STRESS MANAGEMENT

Ultimate Guide to Relieving Stress and Living a Peaceful Life

(Putting Personal Perspectives on Stress Management)

Randall Holland

Published by Tomas Edwards

Stress Management: Ultimate Guide to Relieving Stress and Living a Peaceful Life (Putting Personal Perspectives on Stress Management)

ISBN 978-1-990268-31-1

Legal & Disclaimer

The information contained in this book is not designed to replace or take the place of any form of medicine or professional medical advice. The information in this book has been provided for educational and entertainment purposes only.

The information contained in this book has been compiled from sources deemed reliable, and it is accurate to the best of the Author's knowledge; however, the Author cannot guarantee its accuracy and validity and cannot be held liable for any errors or omissions. Changes are periodically made to this book. You must consult your doctor or get professional medical advice before using any of the suggested remedies, techniques, or information in this book.

Upon using the information contained in this book, you agree to hold harmless the Author from and against any damages, costs, and expenses, including any legal fees potentially resulting from the application of any of the information provided by this guide. This disclaimer applies to any damages or injury caused by the use and application, whether directly or indirectly, of any advice or information presented, whether for breach of contract, tort, negligence, personal injury, criminal intent, or under any other cause of action.

You agree to accept all risks of using the information presented inside this book. You need to consult a professional medical practitioner in order to ensure you are both able and healthy enough to participate in this program.

Table of Contents

Introduction

Stress, no matter how little or how grave, can have a direct impact on your attitude and lifestyle. In fact, it can also have an adverse effect on your body and mind. It is good to identify the reasons behind your stress levels to beat it before it takes you in its grip.

Worries related to academic performance, office work, relationships and finances can perturb you and raise your stress levels while aggravating your physical and mental health.

Stress has become a part of our lives and it is practically impossible to eradicate all stresses completely as they recur time and again with growing responsibilities. However, stress management techniques are effective methods to control stress and resist its influence on our lives.

Frequent headaches, exhaustions, mood swings, sleeplessness etc. are some of the symptoms of stress. If you feel that you are undergoing a stressful life, spend some time with yourself to diagnose the real reasons behind your stress levels.

You can take a break from your hectic life style to find yourself relieved from stress. Stress management is all about taking complete control of your schedule, emotions and thoughts and the way you tackle problems.

Programs on stress management techniques are offered by professionals. These programs are ideal options to deal with your stress levels. In addition, regular exercises, yoga, healthy diet, assertive attitude, focus on priorities, better time management etc. can also work wonders in flushing out stress from various stages of your life.

You need to understand your stresses and deal with them head on. You should try your best to anticipate and prevent problems as much as possible. A positive attitude towards life and spending quality time with family members can also be efficient stress busters.

Stress differs from person to person and hence you need to experiment what can really work for you. A healthy and positive way to deal your stress can enhance your overall wellbeing. The way you feel and deal any stressful situation in life is your choice.

Counselors can only guide you through stress management techniques. They suggest measures to explore positive aspects of life and in confronting situations that arise. Stress management lessons are all about learning when and how to take control.

You can spend leisure hours listening good music or enjoy your hobbies that allow you to counter long term stress and its ill effects. Hobbies help you to refocus and take time for yourself, giving you the chance to fix the stress toll on your mind and body.

Whether you are married or single, a student or working, at home or work, stress challenges might appear irrespective of time or occasion.

A little stress can keep you motivated and focused but when the level increases, it can turn your life into hell. During tough times when you are unable to maintain balance between work and family, inevitable stress might turn out to be real headache.

This guide is fully packed with effective solutions and strategies that can help you discover a new you in you. So control stress before it controls you.

Chapter 1: What Is Stress?

Stress can be defined as the body's way of responding to life's pressures or demands, and it can be caused by either a good or bad experience. What happens is that when change occurs, or something happens in your life, you tend to feel stressed and your body will react by releasing certain chemicals into the blood stream. The chemicals are meant to give you more strength and energy which is actually a good thing if the stress is as a result of physical danger, but dangerous when your stress is in response to an emotional situation. This is so because in physical danger the extra energy and strength can be released, but when it is emotional you won't have an outlet. It is where you find that pile-up of chemicals and energy could lead to chronic stress.

You should also know that whether you are experiencing negative or positive stress, our bodies always have an automatic response. In the body, that response is normally coordinated by a part of the nervous system referred to as the autonomic nervous system and is divided into two, the sympathetic and the parasympathetic. The sympathetic controls the stress response, whereas the parasympathetic controls the relaxation response. In the case of any change or demand, the sympathetic nervous system normally sends messages to different parts of the body – glands, organs and muscles. It is through this that our bodies react and chemicals like cortisol, aldosterone, and adrenaline are released.

These chemicals affect the body in different ways, including increased blood pressure, heart rate, stomach acid build up, blood vessel spasms, and muscle tension, amongst others. As much as these changes are adaptive and may help one to prepare to deal with stress, they can lead to illnesses when the stress is chronic. This is why there is so much emphasis on the importance of stress management, because if it lingers it could lead to chronic diseases. The earlier one alleviates stress the healthier and happier they end up being, and that also reduces the risk of heart problems. The whole idea of stress management involves allowing the parasympathetic nervous system to undo stressful effects and bring about restoration and relaxation in the body.

Most of our stress arises from our fears, worries, regrets, negative perceptions, expectations, and self-criticism. It is important to know that a person's stress level is normally determined more by your perception of the stressor than the stressor itself. This therefore brings us back to the idea of how you react to situations or experiences, no matter how difficult they seem. The truth is all these challenges and difficulties are a part of life, and the more you attach feelings and emotions to them, the more miserable you end up being.

Buddhism teaches us well. It says that nothing is permanent in life and all your difficulties or problems will come to pass. It is thus upon you to make sure that your feelings are not determined by external forces. Learn to let go of all negativity, and this should include replacing negative thoughts with positive ones. Anyone who values their life enough knows that their happiness should always be a priority. This is all about putting in enough effort to find it even in your darkest times. Don't let stress overpower you, as it not only makes you sad but also affects your general health.

Everyone should know that stress is actually a very common problem affecting each person at some point in their lives. Learning how to identify the time you are under stress, the stressor and different ways of coping can highly improve your physical, emotional and mental well-being. All that is encompassed in lessons about stress management which include a spectrum of techniques focused on controlling a person's stress levels, and this is mostly in situations of chronic stress. By effectively managing stress, you will have taken the first step towards improving everyday functioning.

Stress within your comfort zone is not bad, as it helps you perform well under pressure and also motivates you to work harder. When it however becomes overwhelming and prevents you from performing as normal then it becomes a matter of concern. This is mainly because it robs you of your happiness, affects your relationships and productivity. I therefore want you to note that coping with stress effectively, managing it and knowing how to reduce unhealthy stress are very important life skills that we all need. The fact that stress, anxiety and tension are common life problems doesn't mean that you should be ignorant of them or assume they will go away on their own. You will need to take action by finding help and talking to people who can help you.

I hope you now understand what stress really is, and are ready to read more about its management and prevention.

Chapter 2: Sorting Out Your Stressors

The key to getting your life back on track without feeling oppressed by stress is taking control of the stress—before it has a chance to take control of you. The first step in grappling with the stress in your life is sorting out your stressors: figure out precisely which things in your life are stressing you out, which of those things are in your power to change, and which of those things are beyond your control.

What are your stressors?

An important factor in reducing the stress in your life is the ability to identify the things that are causing the stress in your life. Are you going through a major life event, like buying or selling a home? Are you experiencing interpersonal difficulties with a coworker? Are you in serious debt due to credit card usage or medical expenses and struggling to make financial ends meet? Are you a stay-at-home parent feeling frazzled in the face of the various duties that come with parenthood?

These are just a few possibilities on a never-ending list of potential stressors that people might be faced with at any given time—your own list of stressors will be unique to you and your situation.

Make lists

Part of what can make chronic stress feel so insurmountable is the sheer chaos one can feel plunged into when feeling overwhelmed by stress. It can sometimes seem like all the various sources of stress in our lives are like a labyrinth, or a muddled mess of interrelated issues that seem impossible to sort through.

Imagine that your mind is like an old attic, where various baubles and keepsakes and boxes of books have been stowed away for time immemorial. As items continue to be added to the attic for storage, they eventually become cluttered, making it hard to find the one thing you are looking for. Just as with a disorganized and untidy attic, when you are first faced with sorting out your stressors, it can seem to be quite a daunting task. However, by taking things one step at a time and patiently working to organize the clutter that your stress has become, you can start to get a handle on your stressors and get your life back on course. What better way to get organized than to make a list?

List all of your stressors

Take a few moments and think about the roots of the stress you feel. Triggers for the stress you feel should slowly become apparent—and as they do, write them down. Brainstorm and write down every single stressor in your life that you can think of as it comes to the surface of your mind. Once you feel that you have pinpointed all of your various sources of stress, you can move on to compartmentalizing them, by breaking the stressors down into two more lists: one of stressors that are beyond your influence or control, and one of stressors that you can change or work on.

List stressors you have the power to control

Now, you may be saying to yourself, “are you kidding me?! None of these things are in my power to control! That’s why I’m stressed!” But if you look again and pause to give it some thought, you might see that you are not as powerless over your stressors as you think.

Let’s take the example of being in debt. If you are in debt and do not have the financial means to repay your debts and collection agents are calling your house at all hours, you might feel pretty darned helpless. I don’t blame you for feeling overwrought when faced with such a stressful situation. However, it is possible that there are solutions out there that you may have overlooked. Have you checked into debt consolidation programs, or consulted with a personal bankruptcy attorney?

Before deciding that all your stressors belong on the “beyond my control” list, think critically about each one, and ask yourself: "Have I really considered all of the available options?"

Listing the stressors you may have a chance at influencing in a positive way, although challenging, can be very empowering—because it causes you to reexamine your capabilities with regard to enforcing positive changes in your life, and can boost your confidence in your ability to fight back when stress gets tough.

List stressors that are beyond your realm of control

After you have a list of stressors you can change or work on, it's time to focus on making a list of all the stressors you are not able to influence in any way. This is admittedly a rather somber task, because feeling a lack of control over things that are making you miserable is never fun—and outright acknowledging their existence is even less so. However, this is a crucial step in stress management, and as counterintuitive as it may seem—

recognizing and admitting to the things we can't control is the first step in taking control.

Let's consider the case of a stress-inducing major life event, such as buying a new home. Moving is always a stressful experience—that cannot be helped—but what can be helped is how you react to the stress. Instead of allowing yourself to be dragged down into the mire of ruminating on stressful things that are beyond your control, you can vow to focus on the positive aspects of the major life event every time you are tempted to dwell on the negative ones. We will further explore specific strategies for coping with stressors that you cannot control in Chapter 4.

Now that you've made lists of the stressors affecting your quality of life, it's time to put them to use.

Chapter 3: Monitoring Stress

"The truth is that we can learn to condition our minds, bodies, and emotions to link pain or pleasure to whatever we choose. By changing what we link pain and pleasure to, we will instantly change our behaviours."

Anthony Robbins

The first step to manage and handle stress is to realise that you are stressed and detect the early signs of it. Remember, you need to know you are in the distress zone before you can take steps to get out of it.

Early Warning

Here are a number of early warning signals that can act like a trip wire:

Poor emotional control

Excessive moodiness

Exaggerated view towards life

Constant restlessness

Withdrawal from responsibility

Change in appetite or sex drive

Out-of-proportion anxiety

Severe feelings of helplessness

Extreme dependency

Words

Monitoring your conversations and self-talk allows you to estimate your stress level through the language you use. For example the following self-talk must be considered as a sign for further self-examination:

“I feel I am rushing everywhere”

“I can’ relax”

“I feel I have limited room to manoeuvre and I am completely tied up”

“I can’t concentrate anymore, there is so much to do that my attention span is next to nothing”

“I feel sad and hopeless”

Emotions

When stressed, emotions run high and you must stay aware of them:

Overran emotional conversation trips you over.

It is everybody and everything's fault

There is a lot of bickering

There is an overwhelming feeling of fatigue and tiredness

You feel constantly restless and are always worried that more needs to be done

Doors are slammed a little harder, books are dropped on desks, movement is forced a little and the manner is agitated

Body

Your body also provides many useful clues on your stress level, some of these signs include:

Tense body

Near continuous movement or fidgeting, with lots of sitting, walking, back to sitting, almost running and so on.

Tense shoulders

Body fatigue

Use External Help

There are two main ways that you can realise you are ending up distressed. One is by detecting and observing the signs yourself such as those stated above. The other way is to use other people's opinion of you. When you get stressed, other people react to you in certain ways. By observing them and their potential avoidance or cold behaviour you can get more clues about your own state. Stress can be contagious. So others may also show signs of more stress and conflicts are more common in such situations. You can use the other person as a mirror and quickly understand where you are heading.

Friends and family and generally close people can warn you about your stress levels as well. They can see you from a certain point of view that you have no access to and it might be much easier for them to see your transition into the dangerous zone. Naturally, they can take immediate steps to let you know about your stress levels, though they must do this with care. If you are stressed, the last thing you want to here is, "Chill out mate! Why are you so tense?" which may itself trigger the final transition and push you over the edge.

As with all emotions, the best way to get out of one is to do the opposite which in the case of stress means taking steps to become calm and less aroused. If others want to help you, they should do so by using indirect methods which can distract you from what you are stressing about or by removing the source of stress. We will explore a number of techniques later in the course to achieve this.

Daily Log

A great way to monitor your stress levels is to record them systematically.

[illegible]	[illegible]	[illegible]	[illegible]	[illegible]
6:30 AM	Home	Didn't wake up at the time the alarm went off	4	Yoga stretches Planned daily schedule
7:00	Home	Rubbish has not been collected	2	Arrange for extra space to keep the rubbish for next week
7:30	Driveway	Car's side mirror is hit by another car and is broken	3	Happy that the random event was small. It could have been worse. Plan taking car to the garage
9:00	Office	Unexpected auditor visit	4	Rearrange schedule to cope with the unexpected Deep breath Focus
10:00	Office	Have too many emails to drum through	3	It's part of the job. Setup automatic filters to cope with those that are critical first
1:00 PM	Office	Message from garage says that my car is not ready. Need to arrange picking up kids from school	4	Called partner to rearrange based on new circumstances Cancelled a late day meeting to cope with the new schedule Took a walk to reduce stress
6:00	Home	Burned food	2	Used leftover food from the freezer instead

Tension Level: 1 = Minor, 2= Moderate, 3 = Strong, 4 = Excessive

Chapter 4: Types Of Stress

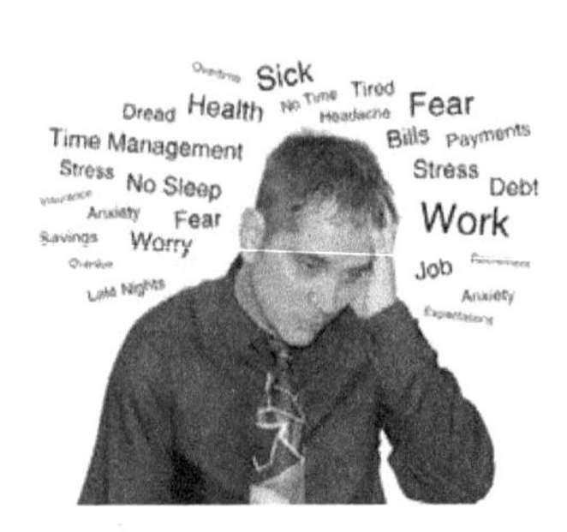

While there is no official list, there are essentially seven different types of stress: mental, professional, physical, chemical, emotional, dietary, and post-traumatic. These are listed in no specific or intentional order, as there is varying degrees and causes for each type. One or two can only afflict some people, while others can have the majority of the list. One type of stress itself can be difficult to manage, but when combined with others, becomes very difficult. Fortunately, we will be able to identify each of these types of stress, and fully understand how and if they affect you.

The first, and most commonly seen type of stress is mental stress. Just about everyone experiences mental stress at some point in their weekly lives, it is only a matter of how much and how severe it can be. Often times, mental stress is self-afflicted, and is caused by issues that do not even exist. For example, let's talk about fear and worry. Fear and worry are not tangible assets. Fear and worry are two items that are made up in the human mind, and only exist to hinder you. Some people have a personality type that makes it near impossible for them not to be anxious or worry constantly.

If you are one of these people, take a few minutes out of your day to do this simple exercise. Sit down with a notebook, and write down all of the things in your day that you believe are causing you anxiety/worry. Make a numbered list of single words, and then turn the page. Do you see a blank sheet of paper? The point of this exercise is that while, yes, there are times in our lives where difficult and cumbersome situations will arise, but the best thing to do is to be strong, and deal with them with a clear head.

It is powerful to believe that you can take a few minutes out of your day just to write down your problems, and turn the page. Of course, this will not solve your problems, or make them go away, but worrying and stressing over small mental situations will not do any good. One of my favorite quotes is “Control what you can control.” Unfortunate things will happen, and difficult situations will arise, but all you can do is face them strong and unburdened by mental stress.

The next type of stress we will be discussing is professional stress. Like mental stress, professional stress is also extremely common, due to the fact that people need to work to live. Professional stress is the most aggravating type of stress, due to the fact many of the issues that cause it are miniscule and not very important, but still happen to be the most annoying of all. A loud co-worker, a rude boss, or the constant burden or strain that comes with your job, among other topics, can cause professional stress. The best way to deal with this type of stress is the "T-chart."

Make a two-column chart, and create two lists. On the left, make a list of unimportant, minuscule things that you can solve or ignore. On the right, make a list of slightly more serious matters, which cannot be solved by pushing under the rug. Remember, stress is caused by your own mind, and how much of it you are forced to deal with is under your control. Is it really worth yelling and angering yourself over the fact that no one cleans up the microwave? Instead of going about your daily routine, change your approach. Maybe put a note on the microwave, post reminders, or call an office meeting. Think of small, yet effective ways you can solve your stressful, everyday problems.

However, we have still not discussed the right side of the t-chart, the more serious matters. Maybe your boss makes rude jokes, or you are constantly harassed by management due to the fact your bus to work is always late. Matters like these can be completely out of your control, as confrontation can lead to you getting reprimanded, and ignoring them can lead to even more stress. Instead of small, short-term fixes to these stressful problems think of bigger, longer-term solutions. If your bus is consistently late, maybe try to arrange a carpool, or save enough money for a small rental car. If your boss is being harassing you, write a letter to management, or try to change your seat in the office. As you can see, not all professional issues can be resolved at the tip of a hat. You must acknowledge that some matters are out of your control, and you have to do your best to make them as pleasant as possible.

The next type of stress we will be evaluating is physical stress. While not as overwhelmingly common as professional or mental stress, it is still a major factor in our society. Physical stress occurs from too much travel, heavy manual labor, or overworking leading to sleep deprivation. Fortunately, many laws and unions have been passed and formed that assist workers in making these types of situations less prevalent. However, they still exist and occur every day. Physical stress is serious due to the fact it can be damaging to your health and well being in the short term. Unlike professional and mental stress, which concerns issues that prolong over a period of time, physical stress takes an immediate toll.

For example, let's say that you worked all through the night, and now have to go back to work in two hours for a full day shift. You will not be very productive, and this lack of sleep can be seriously damaging. Just to put it in perspective, about seven days of no sleep will kill a grown adult. Maybe your back is sore due to the fact your boss made you lift and sort heavy items the previous day. Due to this soreness, you could fall down the stairs, pull a muscle, or sustain a serious injury. Physical stress affects millions of people every day.

The next type of stress we will be discussing is chemical. Chemical stress stems from manufactured consumable goods. Caffeine, tobacco, and any other sort of drug can result in chemical stress. The main reason that chemical stress occurs is dependency, not addiction. Many people interchange these words, not knowing that there is a big difference. Addiction is where your body needs to have a certain substance, to achieve a certain state of mind. Dependency is not as serious as addiction, and only makes your body feel as if it needs a certain substance. Some drugs, such as nicotine and hard drugs, are chemically addictive. You become chemically stressed when your body does not get its "fix" of the substance it craves. Symptoms can include sweating, nervousness, and anxiety, among many other side effects. When someone is chemically stressed, it can become difficult, if not impossible, to accomplish tasks.

Emotional stress is common among people of all ages. When you think of emotional stress, think of the extremes of your emotions. This type of stress stems from prolonged feelings of anger, sadness, depression, etc. One of the most common symptoms of emotional stress is the inability to sleep, or the opposite, sleeping too much. Emotional stress often leads to mood swings, changes in appetite, and conflicting feelings. Like chemical stress, it becomes difficult to do even simple tasks effectively while emotionally stressed.

A common misconception is that only women can truly experience the effects of emotional stress. This is entirely untrue. In fact, it has been found that men are the main victims of extreme emotional stress. Simply because men are taught to keep their emotions in, and act "manly." As you may know, acting like a "man" can mean not showing feelings, and keeping thoughts bottled up. All of this pent up emotion can lead to serious stress and anxiety issues that may not be seen on the surface.

Dietary stress occurs when people are concerned about their weight, when people pressure them about their weight, or when someone has health issues related to being to obese/skinny. By the time an American adult has reached the age of 40, chances are he/she has been involved in at least one dietary fad. Unfortunately, society continually paints the image that the only good male figure is a lean and muscular one, and the only good female figure is a skinny one. Of course, this is not true, and there is beginning to be resistance against this thought process. It is fairly easy to tell if you are afflicted by dietary stress. You might be thinking about food all the time, try to suppress thoughts of hunger, or plan every meal down to the calorie. For some people, they plan out meals and an eating schedule because it is apart of their fitness regimen. But for others, it is due to dietary stress.

Post-traumatic stress (you might know it as Post Traumatic Stress Disorder, or PTSD) is one of the most difficult types of stress to overcome. Post-traumatic stress (we'll refer to it as PTS from now on) occurs when an individual has gone through a mentally horrific or extremely difficult scenario. This kind of stress takes place suddenly and can affect hundreds, thousands, or millions of people all at once. One major example of traumatic stress is the events that occurred on September 11, 2001. As with PTSD, certain everyday events can trigger a reaction.

The events that usually trigger these reactions are significantly emotional, and these kinds of stressors last a long period of time. PTSD can be triggered by any number of stimuli; a car honk, a gunshot, or a loud tapping that reminds an individual of a past experience. This is especially true in the case of war veterans who returned home with the memories of terrible events, only to relive the past traumatic events in their minds at even the slightest trigger.

For common people, PTS can stem from watching someone die, being in a serious car crash, or going through a natural disaster. After experiencing a traumatic event, the said individual will not be able to get the event out of their head. Nightmares, constantly replaying the event in their head, and believing the event will occur again. People who have PTS should see a therapist or mental specialist, as it is not advisable to deal with it on your own, or try to cure your PTS.

Another source of stress for many individuals are major life changes. Major life changes can include deaths, a move, marriages, or children moving out. These types mainly affect adults. When it comes to younger children, a large amount of stress can come from the death of a family member/parent, divorce of loved ones, or a loved one going to prison. To the surprise of many, adolescents are highly affected when people they know go to prison. It is a very foreign concept for many youngsters. It is hard for a young mind to comprehend the fact that someone they know is going to a place where they will not get out of for a long time. You may not recognize this, but when a person experiences happy events they can feel great levels of stress. For example, a professional getting a job promotion can be happy at the new bonuses, but can feel like he/she is under a high level of scrutiny due to the fact the expectation of their performance rises. Marriage is also another great example due to the fact that wedding plannings take a lot of money and time to plan and organize effectively.

Is it possible to have multiple types of stress at once? As you might have guessed, it is entirely possible. When different types of stress are cocktailed together, the results can be not so good. One of the most common combinations is physical and mental stress. They tie in to each other, due to the fact that high levels of brain activity can lead to less sleep, which leads to physical stress. Of course, there are many other combinations, but all can be equally detrimental and harmful to your body and mind.

To wrap up this section, we have to understand that "stress" is not an easily definable item. There are several different types of stress, all with different causes and results. Fortunately, all are treatable, and identifiable. If you ever feel as if your stress is too much to handle, talk to a professional! There are people who go to school and dedicate their careers to helping people who have high levels of stress, and struggle with keeping it under control. While it is admirable to try and cope with stress on your own, it is not always the best decision to keep everything bottled up.

Chapter 5: Body Scan Technique

The body scan technique is a combination of progressive muscle relaxation and breath focus. First, you have to take deep breaths for several minutes. Then, you should start focusing on the different parts of your body. Imagine stress and tension being released from your system. Through this technique, you can increase your awareness of your mind and body connection.

When you practice body scan, see to it that you focus on one area of your body at a time. This way, you can fully concentrate on their details or characteristics. In addition, you have to be objective and neutral. Refrain from making unnecessary judgments or changes.

Clear your mind by taking deep breaths. Inhale slowly and then exhale. Do not rush your breathing. Pause whenever you have to. Let every breath come naturally.

Simply notice the different areas of your body. Do not purposely make any changes. Notice the way your feet feels against the floor or your back against the chair. Notice the sensations that you feel.

Steps on How to Practice the Body Scan Technique

You can begin with your feet. Start with your right foot. Concentrate on your toes and observe how they feel. Observe the way each toe feels against the floor, your other toes, etc. Do not mind the other parts of your body at this time. Just put your full attention towards the toes on your right foot.

Then, you can move to your left foot. Likewise, you should focus on your toes. When you are done, you can observe both of your feet. Observe their temperature. How do they feel?

Move your attention upwards to your ankles. Observe their condition passive. Take deep breaths as you do this. Next, you should move upwards to your legs.

Pay attention to your lower right leg and then to your lower left leg. Observe the way they feel against your clothes, etc.

Scan your knees mentally. Then, move towards your upper legs. Notice them. Observe them in a passive manner. Move your focus to your hips and lower abdomen. Next, you should move your focus to the center of your body. Scan your belly region mentally. Observe how it feels.

Then, you should focus on your back area. Pay attention to the sensations in your middle back and lower back. Scan the sides of your body and your chest. Move your focus towards your arms and then to your hands. You should notice how your fingertips feel. Observe your palms and back of your hands.

Move your focus to your shoulders. Observe how they feel. Are they relaxed? Do you feel tension? Mentally scan your shoulder region and then move towards your neck. Do the same thing. Observe the way your neck and back of your neck feel.

Now, you can move to your head. Focus on the way your entire face feels. Then, you should narrow down your attention to one part of your face at a time. You can start with your chin, cheeks, mouth, nose, ears, and eyes. Then, you can move your focus to your forehead and scalp.

When you are done mentally scanning your head, you can once again mentally scan your entire body. Do not rush this process. Scan your body at a pace that feels comfortable to you. You may linger a few minutes on a particular sensation, but do not get stuck in it.

Once you become completely aware of the way your body feels, you can notice any changes that might have happened. Again, you have to be passive. Take slow and deep breaths as you observe these changes. Afterwards, you should feel more energetic, alert, and awake.

Chapter 6: Having A Heavy Workload Or Too Much Responsibility

Plagued with a heavy workload that's causing you stress? Loosen up and learn how to handle and beat pressure at work from our career pros. We'll share proven workload management tips to help you take over the journey.

Workload Management: Is Your Career at Stake?

In our quick paced period, overwhelming remaining burden is a typical scene. Representatives take more work than they can adapt for different causes. It's because of scaling back, dread of employer stability, or a questionable economy. Further, most organizations intend to meet their objectives and increment their benefits. Laborers regularly observe the need to acknowledge more undertakings and spend longer hours at work.

Why? They most likely need to strike a feeling that they are profitable. Or then again perhaps, these laborers can't decline to their managers. Along these lines, they take more errands, prompting work weight and stress. However, few out of every odd representative takes a gander at overseeing overwhelming outstanding burden a test until something hurtful occurs. That is the reason remaining burden the board is an indispensable ability. Rather than showing you how to perform various tasks, we'll walk you through on the most proficient method to deal with work over-burden effectively.

What is Heavy Workload?

Before sharing the viable remaining burden the board tips, allows first clarify the word overwhelming outstanding task at hand.

To characterize, it implies having more than your necessary remaining burden. For the most part, firms attempt to save money on work expenses and will in general over-burden their laborers. In any case, some simply have harsh fixes in the business leaving them without other decision however to use a little workforce.

How Work Overload Affects Job Performance

What occurs if an organization over-burdens a specialist with an excessive amount of errands? Will it increment the brand's creation rate? Or on the other hand will it strain the laborer and influence the nature of the item? In what ways do the overwhelming outstanding burden influence representatives contrarily? Stress no more! We'll offer the responses to these inquiries.

Now and then, included work doesn't end in expanded degrees of efficiency. Truth be told, it can prompt issues and conditions that decrease an organization's income.

Negative Effects of Too Much Workload?

- Reduced Productivity

- **Stress**
- **Burnout**
- **Mistakes**
- Poor Work-Life Balance

Reduced Productivity: Instead of getting more work accomplished, increased workload results in overwhelmed workers, making them more prone to committing mistakes. Further, overall quality may be at risk, and errors can prompt extra production costs for the firm.

Stress: How does workload cause stress? Often, tired staff members face more stress that may affect their production and cause physical and mental health problems. Stressed employees may not always focus on or tend to their responsibilities. In effect, an excessive workload may cause more issues such as depression and conditions such as high blood pressure.

Burnout: Employees can't take a substantial remaining burden for long in light of the fact that soon unwavering undertakings may cause burnout. In addition, they're inclined to non-appearance, disease, and renunciation. Staff contracting and preparing may get costly for the firm, as well.

Mistakes: The chances of making a mistake may be higher for workers with too many tasks on their plates. Thus, with stress and fatigue, they may overlook safety precautions or miss crucial deadlines that can lead to client loss, decreased revenue, and workplace accidents.

Poor Work-Life Balance: Heavy workload can affect the healthy work-life balance of employees and lead to poor morale and low job satisfaction. In particular, they may become resentful of added tasks and cause workplace apathy.

How to Manage Heavy Workload in Six Easy Ways

How would you adapt to inordinate outstanding task at hand? Do you make to-do agenda before you start? Is utilizing remaining task at hand administration instruments and applications supportive? Notwithstanding how you facilitate your substantial outstanding task at hand, figure out how to deal with the scene. To satisfy every one of your errands, react with the accompanying practices to facilitate your outstanding task at hand in any event, when everything is on top need. Get the undertaking the executives tips beneath.

Pick One Task

Rather than prevalent thinking, performing multiple tasks doesn't give you a chance to complete different errands however makes you slow down one assignment and do another. Thus, rather than beginning everything and completing nothing, pick one occupation and spotlight on it.

Be Positive

In case you're overpowered, odds are, you'll fear taking the necessary steps. To pursue away negative vibes, get siphoned up and energized despite the fact that phony. Be sure on the grounds that the more you do, the more you'll accept and complete it.

Partition It

In the event that a task staggers you, separate it into shorter stages. This training won't just make it increasingly reasonable yet will in like manner help your remaining task at hand arranging and execution.

Set an Alarm

Cut out sufficient opportunity to concentrate on only one errand. Set a caution and expect to complete it before the distributed time closes. When the alert goes off and you're not yet completed, enjoy a reprieve or move to another assignment. This training will make you work more earnestly.

Concentrate on the Next Step

Rather than considering your to be or task as flawless or a success, make it littler in your mind. At the point when you focus on the subsequent stage, you'll understand the work is feasible rather than unthinkable.

Think about a Reason

You'll frequently discover the solidarity to outperform hardships after understanding the explanation you're carrying out a responsibility. Taking a gander at the bigger picture can rouse you to finish it. No compelling reason to identify with some overwhelming outstanding burden cites you see on the web. Utilize these outstanding task at hand administration tips to develop your vocation.

Chapter 7: Causes, Symptoms, And Impact Of Stress

The conduct of research through time produces a common understanding among scholars on the common characteristics of stress though its causes, signs, and impact still vary to date. Scholars agree on the acronym called NUTS. Letter N stands for novelty which in a vernacular language means unique, original or something new. Letter U stands for unpredictability which means something unknown to happen. Letter T stands for threat-to-the-ego which means the perception of incapacity or incompetence. Last is letter S which stands for Sense of Control or less control of the situation if not totally out of control.

Using the principle of NUTS, stress is when we experience something new, that there is no indication as to when or how it will happen and may leave us the perception of incapacity until our body has no control over it. As science continues to expand and build knowledge among us, the word stress evolved and leads to further discoveries. Signs and symptoms of stress were unearthed creating ambiguity on the unpredictability characteristic of stress.

The American Psychological Association (APA) categorized stress according to acute, episodic acute, and chronic. Acute stress is the shortest form of stress and considered not alarming. Acute stress is our reaction to an immediate threat caused by noise, danger, crowding, or isolation. It is the fear of getting hurt or fear of being isolated. Episodic acute stress is common among individuals who are always in a rush and who are into multiple tasking. This stress is caused by one specific event or occurrence. For instance, the feeling of overwhelmed about the number of tasks and has the tendency to worry a lot. Chronic stress, on the other hand, is long term, it occurs over a long period of time. Common causes are financial problems, death of a loved one, divorce and loss of a job.

Causes of stress are classified as external or internal causes according to www.helpguide.org. External causes of stress could be major challenges or event in life like getting divorced or getting married, sudden loss of a job, failing grades in school, discovering the third party in a relationship, overwhelming load of work, family problems and so on. Anything that can happen in your environment affecting the level of your adrenalin or leaves you with that sense of feeling which you have little control of are considered external stressor. Your pet, the food you eat, and your electronic gadgets can be the external stressor considering that those should be a stress reliever instead. Hence, anything in our environment, being external to the human body is a stressor. Internal causes of stress, on the other hand, are too much negativity, failure to accept uncertainty or denial of facts, manner of thinking, not being flexible and too many expectations.

Scott (2019) wrote an article identifying the major causes of stress, hence causes of stress are also categorized from the perspective of major and minor. Among the major causes she identified are financial problems, work, personal relationship, parenting, daily life, personality, and resources. The rest belong to the minor causes of stress.

The Australian government, thru their health direct website, identified the causes of stress according to major life events, routine stress, traumatic stress, and other causes. Financial issues are considered as one primary cause of stress among Australians. Life events can be positive and negative events. Getting married or having a child are life events. Routine stress is what you experience in daily life or has something to do with your daily routine from the time you wake up in the morning until you went up to bed on the same day. Cleaning the house, interaction with friends, going to school and the food you eat can be part of your routine stress. Accidents or being subjective to extreme circumstances are an example of traumatic stress.

Symptoms or signs of stress varies, depending on the individual's capacity to handle stressor. It can manifest through behavior or emotions, physical and in the cognitive ability of an individual. Emotional symptoms of stress can be crying, sadness, fear and fuming. Physical symptoms of stress can be uneasiness, dizziness, stomach pains, vomiting, insomnia, allergies, coldness and more. There are also signs manifested in the cognitive ability of individuals, such as loss of track, difficulty in remembering, constant worrying and inability to decide or focus. An individual under or experiencing stress can pretend or deny the fact but stress always find its way out in the human body. Chronic stress can lead to death.

The American Institute of Stress (AIS) listed 50 common signs and symptoms of stress. Top of their list is the frequent headaches or pain while the last item is the impulse buying. Interesting to see in the list apart from the impulsive buying are the following symptoms: flatulence, goosebumps, and belching. Take note that in medical science flatulence is considered good for health and belching is a sign of fullness in the stomach. Impulse buying is a woman common behavior and goosebumps is usually associated with admiration for something extraordinary. If you are experiencing those, which I guess all of us did, it may not harm to look and see if that is not a sign of stress after all.

Since most if not all have common knowledge on the common signs and symptoms of stress, let us look at some of the peculiar signs or the uncommon symptoms of stress. Dissociating stress from the common things that we normally do, from those that we thought part of our daily routine and from those that are common to our friends, family and to the community is a bit tricky and fiddly. Stress needs medical attention, but the following symptoms or sign will give you a second thought. Here are some of the odds signs of stress:

Feeling thirsty. Who would think that when you feel thirsty there is a probability that you are experiencing stress? The culprit is the small glands located in your kidney, on top of the kidney to be precise. Gratis to the medical world for locating every single gland in our body and their countless research to understand their functions. According to the study, that small glands in your kidney can initiate or start pumping out stress hormones into the human body in the sudden surge of adrenalin.

Falling hair. Hair just falls out over time by simply brushing or washing it, because falling hair is normal. According to the American Academy of Dermatology, shedding between 50 and 100 strands of hair a day is normal. Excessive hair shedding however of more than a hundred, should you opted to count your falling hair, is a condition called telogen effluvium. Any stressful event like losing or breaking up in a relationship can cause androgens hormones to spike affecting hair follicles that can lead to temporary hair loss. Premature graying of hair unless genetically linked is also associated with stress. By the way, be careful to dissociate falling hair from hair loss, the former is different from the latter.

Napping or feeling sleepy. We have a common habit of taking a short nap, in the afternoon, in between work or when the atmosphere induces it. We do this to relieve fatigue, to rejuvenate and to put the brain to rest. However, according to study frequent napping is a sign of stress. How ironic that we are considering a nap as a stress reliever and yet it is also stressing itself. According to medical science, one symptom of depression is oversleeping.

Fawning or being submissive. When a person is subjected to an argument, there are those who would choose to submit or cooperate in order to avoid further conflict or simply to stop any conflict and move on. However, Dr. Curtis Reisinger of the Zucker Hillside Hospital said that fawning is a less-recognized stress response. It comes whenever a person withholds the emotions to stop or to avoid conflict.

Odd dreams. We experienced waking up at night crying because we dreamt something bad. Without stress, dreams usually get progressively more positive as you sleep, so you wake up in a better mood than you were in when you went to bed, says Rosalind Cartwright, Ph.D., an emeritus professor of psychology at Rush University Medical Center. But when a person is under stress, the tendency is to wake up more often, thereby disrupting the process and allowing unpleasant imagery to recur all night. Recurring dreams can make you think and affect you mentally–especially if they're upsetting–but even if they aren't. Bizarre dreams can make you feel tired and on edge, which ultimately impacts other areas of your life, like work and family.

Breakouts and acne. According to science, acne or breakouts are part of growing out. Hormones known as androgens increases causing the sebaceous glands to enlarge and make more sebum during the puberty stage of both male and female. Hormonal changes related to pregnancy can affect sebum production and result in breakouts. Some allergic reactions to food or too much gluten in our food can cause acne. White bread can also cause acne. Stress can increase inflammation leading to breakouts, according to the dermatology professor of Wake Forest University.

Muscle twitching. Muscle twitching around the eyes is connected to your stress level though doctors still aren't sure why. According to the Mayo Clinic, stress can cause eyelid spasms. While twitching isn't painful, it annoying, distracting and sometimes alarming depending on the frequency and length of occurrence.

Twitching can be for a few minutes or may take several months before it is gone.

Common colds or flu. Colds and flu are normally associated with the sudden change in temperature, change of climate or getting infected through friends, in school, and within the family. But getting colds because of stress may seems unlikely. According to the study, getting sick more than the average person and your body catching virus easily can be caused by stress. Stress hormones can also attack the immune system the way it affects the human nervous system.

Not feeling well (Unknown disease). Each disease has its own signs and symptoms, but what if a person is exhibiting signs and symptoms of a disease and yet your body or organ is perfectly normal. Urination problem is normally associated with kidney and diabetes, however, after several tests, results are normal and nothing to worry about. There is also the feeling that you are unwell, but you cannot identify exactly what it is. Stress hormones are incredibly impossible sometimes.

Sugar cravings. Mostly treated as comfort foot but ironically considered as a sign of stress. Who can say no to sweets? We love to eat, and sugar is almost everywhere in the food we eat daily. People become accustomed to it including our body, our system. If cravings for sugar is associated with stress, what else is not?

While we look at stress in a purely negative sense, there are times when stress is also beneficial to us for the simple reason that it encourages an individual to meet a deadline or get things done. It pushes our self to determine our capacity or limits as a person. Stress also serves as a means or way to discover talent and pursue an individual passion in life. Let's proceed with the discussion.

Like classifying the causes of stress, the signs and symptoms of stress can be endless and may evolve thru times. Both the causes and the symptoms are congruent with the changing or evolving human environment. As technology progresses, it created or developed a new kind of stressor. We initially acknowledged that anything and everything around us can be a stressor depending on how we deal with it or depending our individual capacity to deal with it. But while new discoveries and breakthrough are good in the world of science, they add up to the list of potential stressors.

The impact of stress can be seen in your body, your thoughts and feelings, and your behavior. According to the mayoclinic.org the common impact of stress in the body are fatigue, headache, change in sex drive and stomach upset among others. In thoughts or mood, it could be irritability, lack of focus, overwhelmed and sadness. Effects on behavior on the hand could be over/less eating, social withdrawal, alcohol or drug misuse.

The AIS looks at the impact of stress using the body systems, the cardiovascular system, the digestive system, the immune system, the muscular system, and the central nervous system. For instance, whenever we encounter fear, the brain that is connected with the nervous system (CNS) gets hypothalamus to tell the adrenal glands to release the stress hormones adrenaline and cortisol. These hormones then increase the heartbeat and send blood rushing to the areas that need it most in an emergency, such as your muscles (defense mechanism) and heart. The rush of hormones can upset your digestive system and likely to produce heartburn or acid reflux. Stress doesn't cause ulcers but can cause existing ulcers to act up. When the perceived fear is gone, the hypothalamus should tell all systems to go back to normal. If the CNS fails to return to normal, or if the stressor doesn't go away, the response will continue.

Interestingly, the AIS also mentioned that while short-term stress tends to produce more male hormone testosterone the effect doesn't last. The man's testosterone levels begin to drop in a prolonged stress condition. Stress can interfere with sperm production and cause erectile dysfunction or impotence. Stress for women can lead to irregular, heavier, or more painful periods and can magnify the physical symptoms of menopause.

Causes, Symptoms, and Impact of Stress

The acronym of stress is called NUTS. This means stress is unique or has novelty, it is unpredictable, it is a threat to the ego and sense of control is compromised.

Stress can be categorized as acute, episodic acute, and chronic, depending on its impact on the human body.

Stress has been so ingrained in the people's daily life, it could easily be associated with your pet, eating food and the electronic system.

Causes of stress can be categorized as internal or external and major or minor causes.

There 50are common signs and symptoms of stress. Interesting to note are the following symptoms: flatulence, goosebumps, belching and impulse buying.

Some of the peculiar signs or the uncommon of symptoms of stress are being thirsty, falling hair, napping, fawning, odd dreams, common colds, muscle twitching, unknown disease, and sugar cravings.

Stress is also beneficial to us for the simple reason that it encourages an individual to meet a deadline or get a task done. It also serves as a means or way to discover talent and pursue an individual passion in life.

Impact of stress can be harmful to the body system, the cardiovascular system, the digestive system, the immune system, the muscular system, and the central nervous system.

Stress doesn't cause ulcers but can cause existing ulcers to act up.

Stress can interfere with sperm production and cause erectile dysfunction or impotence.

Chapter 8: Stop Overthinking Will Set You Free From Anxiety

What holds people back from the life they really want to live? I would say that the average person does not know how to stop overthinking. They can overcome most small problems, until those problems become so great (from their own thoughts overpowering reality or some outside circumstance changes to make them bigger) and they cannot handle them any longer.

We overthink favorable stuff until they no longer look so favorable - and that's exactly when stress and anxiety begin to develop. Or you might overanalyze and deconstruct things. Trusting things will be ok is a great thing. Getting lost in a kind of rethinking disorder can lead to getting stuck in life and you unintentionally sabotaging the good aspects that exist in life.

I understand that. I understand. I used to think about things a lot, and it took all the fun out of my existence. In the last ten years or so, I figured out how work with my thoughts and learn how to manage my stress by ceasing to overthink every single thing. So now, I know what to do to defeat this negative and unproductive and life sucking process.

In this section, I would like to share 12 habits that helped me in a big, big way to become a much more straightforward and creative thinker and lead a happier and less fearful life.

1. Look at things in a broader point of view.

It is extremely easy to get to a place where you feel like you've fallen into a trap of overthinking small things in life. When you find yourself overthinking something, ask yourself: Will this matter in 5 years? And even in 5 weeks?

I've found that broadening the viewpoint by using this easy method can rapidly snap me out of overthinking and help me to let go of that circumstance. It helps me cease overthinking about the issue and helps me focus my time and energy on something else that, in fact, does matter to me.

2. Set quick time-limits for decisions.

If you do not have a time-limit for when you must make a choice and take action, then you can just keep turning your ideas around and around in your head and view them from all angles in your mind for a very long time. So you must begin making choices and spring into action by setting deadlines in your everyday life. No matter if it's a small or larger decision.

Here's what has actually worked for me:

For little decisions, like, preparing meals, respond to an e- mail, or workout, I typically allow myself 30 seconds or less to make a choice. For larger or more important decisions that would have taken me days or weeks to make a decision about in the past, I allow myself 30 minutes to decide, and no longer than the rest of the workday to make a decision.

3.Stop setting your day up for stress and overthinking. You can't completely avoid exceptionally hard or frustrating days. But, you can minimize them in your month and year by getting a great start to your day and by not setting yourself up for unnecessary stress, suffering, and overthinking.

Three things that help me:

a) Get a good start:

I've discussed this often at this point. Due to the fact that how you begin your day tends to set the tone for your day. A stressed early morning leads to a frazzled day. Consuming undesirable information during the day as you work at your daily tasks tends to cause more cynical ideas throughout the rest of your day. While for instance, reading something positive over breakfast, getting some exercise, and then getting started with your most vital task of the day - sets an excellent tone for the day and will help you to remain positive.

b) Do a single-task and take regular breaks:

This will assist you to keep a sharp focus throughout your day and to get what's vital done while also enabling you to rest and recharge, so you don’t get frazzled. And this calms the mind. With the narrow focus you can think clearly and decisively, thus preventing you from ending up in a worried and overthinking headspace.

c) Decrease your everyday input:

Excessive information, for example, spending time reviewing your inbox, perusing Facebook, or your Twitter account, or examining how your blog site or website is doing triggers more input and mess in your mind as your day progresses. Therefore it ends up being more difficult to think in a simple and clear way and makes it easier for you to lapse back into that familiar overthinking practice.

4. Become a person of action:

When you comprehend how to get started with finding a solution for your every day problems, then you'll hesitate less and, as a result, overthink less.

Setting due dates for things and creating an excellent tone for the day are two things that have helped me tremendously to become a lot more of a person of action. Taking little actions forward and just focusing on getting one thing done at a time is another practice that has, worked exceptionally.

It works so well because you do not feel overwhelmed. Therefore, you will cease having the urge to run away into procrastination or lazy inactiveness.

And in spite of the fact that you may be reluctant, taking simple actions is a small thing you can do to keep yourself from getting disabled in fear.

5.Understand that you can not control everything: Obsessing over things 50 times over, can be an approach to attempt to manage everything. To cover every possibility, so you do not risk making a mistake, stop working, or looking foolish. However, you must understand you simply cannot control everything and you have to act in making decisions about everyday life. Everyone who inspires you has made mistakes, because everyone does. Those people take action, make decisions and then accept the outcome of their choices. These inspirational people use all of their choices, the good and bad ones, as an opportunity to learn and grow. Those things that may look undesirable have, in fact, taught them a lot and have really been important to assist them in growing.

Stop trying to manage everything. Given the fact that no one can see all possible situations beforehand, attempting to do so simply does not work.

This is naturally a lot easier said than done. Work on this technique little by little until it becomes more comfortable for you.

6.Train your mind to cease overthinking - especially at times when the mind is not the sharpest:

In the past, when I was extremely hungry or tired and was my mind was not the sharpest - I would try to go to sleep and have unfavorable ideas buzzing around in my mind.

In the past, they might have overwhelmed me and kept me from falling asleep, or my unfocused mind became frustrated because it was not sharpe due to the fact I was tired - and not the optimum time to make any important decisions.

Nowadays, I've become good at capturing them rapidly and to state to myself: No, no, we are not going to think about this right now. I understand that when I'm starving or sleepy, then my mind often tends to be unfocused or unclear and also prone to negativeness. So I follow up my "no, no ..." expression, and I say to myself that I will contemplate this issue when I have eaten or gotten some much needed rest and my mind will work better - after I've eaten, or in the morning after I have gotten my rest.

It took a bit of practice to get this to work, but I've gotten quite proficient at postponing thinking in this way. When I review a scenario with some level-headed thinking, then in

80% of the cases, the concern is truly small to nonexistent, and, from experience, I understand this truth. And if there is a time sensitive or urgent issue, then my mind is prepared to handle it in a better and more useful way.

7. Do not get lost in vague worries;

Getting lost in unclear fears about a circumstance in my life is another trap I've often fallen under, that has stimulated overthinking.. My mind would run wild imagining a possible future disastrous situation that might occur.

So I've learned to ask myself: honestly, what is the worst that could happen?

B025

And when I figure out what the worst that could occur actually is then, I can then spend a little time to contemplating what I can do if that unlikely thing happens. I've found that the worst that could realistically happen is normally something that is not as scary as what my fearful mind might produce. Finding clearness in this way normally just takes a couple of minutes and a bit of energy, and it can conserve you a lot of time and suffering.

8. Work out:

This may sound a little different. Working out can help to let go of internal stress and worries. It most frequently makes me feel more decisive, and when I was more of an over thinker, it was often my go-to technique of changing my headspace into a more positive one.

9. Get Adequate Good Quality Sleep:

When it comes to keeping a positive mindset and not getting lost in unfavorable ideas, I think this is one of the most frequently overlooked, and one of the most important components.

When you have not slept enough you are more susceptible to getting lost in unclear fears about life circumstances. You become far more susceptible to fretting and pessimism. You begin thinking far less clearly than you would otherwise with adequate sleep. Without enough quality sleep, you will get lost in thoughts going around and around in your mind, painfully overthinking, and with a lack of clarity.

Let me share a couple of my favorite pointers that assist me to sleep much better:

a) Keep it cool.

It can feel good in the beginning to get into a warm bedroom. However, I've discovered that I sleep better and more calmly with less unpleasant dreams if I keep the bedroom cool.

b) Keep the earplugs close by.

If you, like me, are easily woken up by noises, then a simple pair of earplugs can be a life-saver! These affordable products have actually helped me to get an excellent night's sleep and sleep through snorers, loud cats, and other disruptions more times than I can count!

c) Don’t force yourself to go to bed if you are not tire:

If you don't feel sleepy, don't go to bed just because its quote on quote time to go to bed. In my experience, forcing myself to try to go to bed when I’m not tired just allows an hour or more to turn and flip in bed overthinking because I’m unable to fall asleep. A better solution in these scenarios is to wind down for an additional 20-30 minutes on the sofa with, for instance, some reading. This assists me to go to sleep faster and, in the end, get more sleep.

10. Spend more of your time in the present moment:

By getting and staying in the present moment in your everyday life rather than living in the past or consuming your thoughts on the future you can replace the time you typically invest in overthinking things with simply being right here right now. Three techniques I often use to reconnect with the present moment:

a) Slow down.

Each day consciously move slower, talk slower, walk slower. By doing so, you become more conscious of how you use your body and what is happening all around you; in the moment. Tell yourself: Now I am ... I often inform myself this: Now I am X. And X might be brushing my teeth and walking in the woods and or preparing a meal.

That quick tip helps my mind stop wandering and return my attention to what's going on at this minute.

b) Reconnect:

When you feel lost in overthinking, then interrupt the thought by— in your mind—

screaming to yourself: STOP! Reconnect with the present moment by taking only 1-2 minutes to concentrate on what's currently happening around you fully. With all the senses, take it all in. Feel it, listen to it, taste it, see it, and fully connect it in your mind and body.

11. Spend much more time with people who don't overthink things:

Your social environment plays a huge part in your mental

state. And not simply the individuals and groups close to you in your personal life. Also, what you read, listen to, and watch—blog sites, books, online forums, movies, podcasts, and music you consume or read or listen to. Consider if there are any sources in your life that tend to encourage or instigate you overthinking. And consider what individuals or sources have the opposite impact on you - those things that help you relax or be more present.

Find ways to spend more of your time and attention with individuals and avenues that have a positive impact on your thinking and less on the influences that tend to enhance you to overthink.

12. Be conscious of your problems:

Knowing what's bothering you is crucial to break the habit of overthinking. However, if you believe that you'll simply remember to stop overthinking throughout your typical day, then you're most likely simply fooling yourself. Because I consciously work on this process daily, it has become natural for me and I have developed a few pointers. The most helpful thing is to put a note on the whiteboard I have on my wall at home. It states, "Keep things very simple." Seeing this a couple of times throughout my day motivates me to snap out more easily from overthinking and to reduce this negative behavior over time.

Two other tips that you can use:

A small hand written note. Merely use a post-it note or something similar and jot down expressions, a question like "Am I overcomplicating this?" or some other pointer that appeals to you. Put that note where you can easily see it For instance, on your bedside table, your restroom mirror, or next to your computer screen.

A suggestion on your smartphone. Jot down among the expressions above, or one of your own choosing in a pointer app on your mobile phone. For instance, I use my Android phone, and the totally free app called Google Keep to do this.

Last Thought.

Trying to manage all the outcomes of your life is undoubtedly the primary cause of frustration and overthinking. You are likewise doomed to feverishly overthink about what to do in every minute of your life in fear of what might, as a result, occur next because when you do. The very best thing you can do is to persuade yourself not to overthink. Understand that you have no say in what takes place in your life, and that it is of no benefit to you to fret about it. The universe has your fate decided, so you need to just make the most of every moment. Work to understand this prior to anything you might be thinking twice to do, and it'll assist you to stop overthinking and just act, choose.

Another thing you can do - make particular time frames to make a decision about something you need to act on. Whether it is to talk to someone or go visit somebody or more significant life choices, which may be causing you to overthink; take a minute for the small, less important decisions, and a couple of days, at most, for the bigger ones in life. This will propel you to assess a decision rationally and research to make the best choice possible, in a timely manner. Once you do make a choice, immediately act on that choice and don't second guess yourself. It may be frightening, but you'll find it rewarding in time.

At the end of the day, we are all capable of achieving all the things we have dreamed of, and the only thing we have to do is to steer ourselves in the right direction, trust ourselves and eliminate our deterrents. And that will make all the difference.

Chapter 9: Stress Symptoms, Signs, And Causes

Improving Your Ability to Handle Stress

Stress isn't always bad. In small doses, it can help you perform under pressure and motivate you to do your best. But when you're constantly running in emergency mode, your mind and body pay the price. If you frequently find yourself feeling frazzled and overwhelmed, it's time to take action to bring your nervous system back into balance. You can protect yourself—and improve how you think and feel—by learning how to recognize the signs and symptoms of chronic stress and taking steps to reduce its harmful effects.

What Is Stress?

Stress is your body's way of responding to any kind of demand or threat. When you sense danger—whether it's real or imagined—the body's defenses kick into high gear in a rapid, automatic process known as the "fight-or-flight" reaction or the "stress response."

The stress response is the body's way of protecting you. When working properly, it helps you stay focused, energetic, and alert. In emergency situations, stress can save your life—giving you extra strength to defend yourself, for example, or spurring you to slam on the brakes to avoid a car accident.

Stress can also help you rise to meet challenges. It's what keeps you on your toes during a presentation at work, sharpens your concentration when you're attempting the game-winning free throw, or drives you to study for an exam when you'd rather be watching TV. But beyond a certain point, stress stops being helpful and starts causing major damage to your health, mood, productivity, relationships, and your quality of life.

Fight-Or-Flight Response: What Happens In The Body

When you feel threatened, your nervous system responds by releasing a flood of stress hormones, including adrenaline and cortisol, which rouse the body for emergency action. Your heart pounds faster, muscles tighten, blood pressure rises, breath quickens, and your senses become sharper. These physical changes increase your strength and stamina, speed up your reaction time, and enhance your focus—preparing you to either fight or flee from the danger at hand.

The Four Common Types of Stress

Dr. Karl Albrecht, a management consultant and conference speaker based in California, is a pioneer in the development of stress-reduction training for businesspeople. He defined four common types of stress in his 1979 book, "Stress and the Manager."

Albrecht's four common types of stress are:

1. Time stress.

2. Anticipatory stress.

3. Situational stress.

4. Encounter stress.

Let's look at each of these types of stress in detail, and discuss how you can identify and deal with each one.

1. Time Stress

You experience time stress when you worry about time, or the lack thereof. You worry about the number of things that you have to do, and you fear that you'll fail to achieve something important. You might feel trapped, unhappy, or even hopeless.

Common examples of time stress include worrying about deadlines or rushing to avoid being late for a meeting.

Managing Time Stress

Time stress is one of the most common types of stress that we experience today. It is essential to learn how to manage this type of stress if you're going to work productively in a busy organization.

First, learn good time management skills. This can include using To-Do Lists or if you have to manage many simultaneous projects, Action Programs.

Next, make sure that you're devoting enough time to your important priorities. Unfortunately, it's easy to get caught up in seemingly urgent tasks which actually have little impact on your overall objectives. This can leave you feeling exhausted, or feeling that you worked a full day yet accomplished nothing meaningful.

Your important tasks are usually the ones that will help you reach your goals, and working on these projects is a better use of your time. Our article on Eisenhower's Urgent/Important Principle explains how to balance urgent and important tasks, and our article on prioritization helps you separate tasks that you need to focus on from those you can safely put off.

If you often feel that you don't have enough time to complete all of your tasks, learn how to create more time in your day. This might mean coming in early or working late so that you have quiet time to focus. You should also use your peak working time to concentrate on your most important tasks – because you're working more efficiently, this helps you do more with the time you have.

For instance, if you're a morning person, schedule the tasks that need the greatest concentration during this time. Our article "Is This a Morning Task " helps you learn how to prioritize your tasks and schedule them during your most productive times of day. You can leave less important tasks, like checking email, for times when your energy levels drop.

Also, make sure that you're polite but assertive about saying "no" to tasks that you don't have the capacity to do.

2. Anticipatory Stress

Anticipatory stress describes stress that you experience concerning the future. Sometimes this stress can be focused on a specific event, such as an upcoming presentation that you're going to give. However, anticipatory stress can also be vague and undefined, such as an overall sense of dread about the future, or a worry that "something will go wrong."

Managing Anticipatory Stress

Because anticipatory stress is future based, start by recognizing that the event you're dreading doesn't have to play out as you imagine. Use positive visualization techniques to imagine the situation going right.

Research shows that your mind often can't tell the difference, on a basic neurological level, between a situation that you've visualized going well repeatedly and one that's actually happened.

3. Situational Stress

You experience situational stress when you're in a scary situation that you have no control over. This could be an emergency. More commonly, however, it's a situation that involves conflict, or a loss of status or acceptance in the eyes of your group. For instance, getting laid off or making a major mistake in front of your team are examples of events that can cause situational stress.

Managing Situational Stress

Situational stress often appears suddenly, for example, you might get caught in a situation that you completely failed to anticipate. To manage situational stress better, learn to be more self-aware. This means recognizing the "automatic" physical and emotional signals that your body sends out when you're under pressure.

For example, imagine that the meeting you're in suddenly dissolves into a shouting match between team members. Your automatic response is to feel a surge of anxiety. Your stomach knots and feels bloated. You withdraw into yourself and, if someone asks for your input, you have a difficult time knowing what to say.

Conflict is a major source of situational stress. Learn effective conflict resolution skills, so that you're well-prepared to handle the stress of conflict when it arises. It's also important to learn how to manage conflict in meetings since resolving group conflict can be different from resolving individual issues.

Everyone reacts to situational stress differently, and it's essential that you understand both the physical and emotional symptoms of this stress, so that you can manage them appropriately. For instance, if your natural tendency is to withdraw emotionally, then learn how to think on your feet and communicate better during these situations. If your natural response is to get angry and shout, then learn how to manage your emotions.

4. Encounter Stress

Encounter stress revolves around people. You experience encounter stress when you worry about interacting with a certain person or group of people – you may not like them, or you might think that they're unpredictable.

Encounter stress can also occur if your role involves a lot of personal interactions with customers or clients, especially if those groups are in distress. For instance, physicians and social workers have high rates of encounter stress, because the people they work with routinely don't feel well, or are deeply upset.

This type of stress also occurs from "contact overload": when you feel overwhelmed or drained from interacting with too many people.

Managing Encounter Stress

Because encounter stress is focused entirely on people, you'll manage this type of stress better by working on your people skills. To find out how good your people skills are take our quiz, and discover the areas that you need to develop.

A good place to start is to develop greater emotional intelligence. Emotional intelligence is the ability to recognize the emotions, wants, and needs of yourself and of others. This is an important skill in interacting with others and in building good relationships.

It's also important to know when you're about to reach your limit for interactions in the day. Everyone has different symptoms for encounter stress, but a common one is withdrawing psychologically from others and working mechanically. Another common symptom is getting cranky, cold, or impersonal with others in your interactions. When you start to experience these symptoms, do whatever you can to take a break. Go for a walk, drink water, and practice deep breathing exercises.

Empathy is a valuable skill for coping with this type of stress, because it allows you to see the situation from the other person's perspective. This gives you greater understanding and helps you to structure your communications so that you address the other person's feelings, wants, and needs

The Effects Of Chronic Stress

Your nervous system isn't very good at distinguishing between emotional and physical threats. If you're super stressed over an argument with a friend, a work deadline, or a mountain of bills, your body can react just as strongly as if you're facing a true life-or-death situation. And the more your emergency stress system is activated, the easier it becomes to trigger, making it harder to shut off.

If you tend to get stressed out frequently, like many of us in today's demanding world, your body may exist in a heightened state of stress most of the time. And that can lead to serious health problems. Chronic stress disrupts nearly every system in your body. It can suppress your immune system, upset your digestive and reproductive systems, increase the risk of heart attack and stroke, and speed up the aging process. It can even rewire the brain, leaving you more vulnerable to anxiety, depression, and other mental health problems.

Health problems caused or exacerbated by stress include:

1. Depression and anxiety
2. Pain of any kind
3. Sleep problems
4. Autoimmune diseases
5. Digestive problems
6. Skin conditions, such as eczema
7. Heart disease
8. Weight problems
9. Reproductive issues
10. Thinking and memory problems

Signs And Symptoms Of Stress Overload

The most dangerous thing about stress is how easily it can creep up on you. You get used to it. It starts to feel familiar, even normal. You don't notice how much it's affecting you, even as it takes a heavy toll. That's why it's important to be aware of the common warning signs and symptoms of stress overload.

Cognitive symptoms:

- Memory problems
- Inability to concentrate
- Poor judgment
- Seeing only the negative
- Anxious or racing thoughts
- Constant worrying

Emotional symptoms:

- Depression or general unhappiness
- Anxiety and agitation
- Moodiness, irritability, or anger
- Feeling overwhelmed
- Loneliness and isolation
- Other mental or emotional health problems

Physical symptoms:

- Aches and pains
- Diarrhea or constipation
- Nausea, dizziness

- Chest pain, rapid heart rate
- Loss of sex drive
- Frequent colds or flu

Behavioral symptoms:

- Eating more or less
- Sleeping too much or too little
- Withdrawing from others
- Procrastinating or neglecting responsibilities
- Using alcohol, cigarettes, or drugs to relax
- Nervous habits (e.g. nail-biting, pacing)

Causes Of Stress

The situations and pressures that cause stress are known as stressors. We usually think of stressors as being negative, such as an exhausting work schedule or a rocky relationship. However, anything that puts high demands on you can be stressful. This includes positive events such as getting married, buying a house, going to college, or receiving a promotion.

Of course, not all stress is caused by external factors. Stress can also be internal or self-generated, when you worry excessively about something that may or may not happen, or have irrational, pessimistic thoughts about life.

Finally, what causes stress depends, at least in part, on your perception of it. Something that's stressful to you may not faze someone else; they may even enjoy it. While some of us are terrified of getting up in front of people to perform or speak, for example, others live for the spotlight. Where one person thrives under pressure and performs best in the face of a tight deadline, another will shut down when work demands escalate. And while you may enjoy helping to care for your elderly parents, your siblings may find the demands of caretaking overwhelming and stressful.

Common external causes of stress include:

- Major life changes
- Work or school
- Relationship difficulties
- Financial problems
- Being too busy
- Children and family

Common internal causes of stress include:

- Pessimism
- Inability to accept uncertainty
- Rigid thinking, lack of flexibility
- Negative self-talk
- Unrealistic expectations / perfectionism
- All-or-nothing attitude

Top 10 Stressful Life Events

According to the widely validated Holmes and Rahe Stress Scale, these are the top ten stressful life events for adults that can contribute to illness:

1. Death of a spouse

2. Divorce

3. Marriage separation

4. Imprisonment

5. Death of a close family member

6. Injury or illness

7. Marriage

8. Job loss

9. Marriage reconciliation

10. Retirement

What's Stressful For You?

Whatever event or situation is stressing you out, there are ways of coping with the problem and regaining your balance. Some of life's most common sources of stress include:

- Stress at work

While some workplace stress is normal, excessive stress can interfere with your productivity and performance, impact your physical and emotional health, and affect your relationships and home life. It can even determine the difference between success and failure on the job. Whatever your ambitions or work demands, there are steps you can take to protect yourself from the damaging effects of stress, improve your job satisfaction, and bolster your well-being in and out of the workplace.

- Job loss and unemployment stress

Losing a job is one of life's most stressful experiences. It's normal to feel angry, hurt, or depressed, grieve for all that you've lost, or feel anxious about what the future holds. Job loss and unemployment involves a lot of change all at once, which can rock your sense of purpose and self-esteem. While the stress can seem overwhelming, there are many steps you can take to come out of this difficult period stronger, more resilient, and with a renewed sense of purpose.

- Caregiver stress

The demands of caregiving can be overwhelming, especially if you feel that you're in over your head or have little control over the situation. If the stress of caregiving is left unchecked, it can take a toll on your health, relationships, and state of mind — eventually leading to burnout. However, there are plenty of things you can do to rein in the stress of caregiving and regain a sense of balance, joy, and hope in your life.

- Grief and loss

Coping with the loss of someone or something you love is one of life's biggest stressors. Often, the pain and stress of loss can feel overwhelming. You may experience all kinds of difficult and unexpected emotions, from shock or anger to disbelief, guilt, and profound sadness. While there is no right or wrong way to grieve, there are healthy ways to cope with the pain that, in time, can ease your sadness and help you come to terms with your loss, find new meaning, and move on with your life.

How Much Stress Is Too Much?

Because of the widespread damage stress can cause, it's important to know your own limit. But just how much stress is "too much" differs from person to person. Some people seem to be able to roll with life's punches, while others tend to crumble in the face of small obstacles or frustrations. Some people even thrive on the excitement of a high-stress lifestyle.

Factors that influence your stress tolerance level include:

- Your support network: A strong network of supportive friends and family members is an enormous buffer against stress. When you have people you can count on, life's pressures don't seem as overwhelming. On the flip side, the lonelier and more isolated you are, the greater your risk of succumbing to stress.

- Your sense of control: If you have confidence in yourself and your ability to influence events and persevere through challenges, it's easier to take stress in stride. On the other hand, if you believe that you have little control over your life—that you're at the mercy of your environment and circumstances—stress is more likely to knock you off course.

- Your attitude and outlook: The way you look at life and its inevitable challenges makes a huge difference in your ability to handle stress. If you're generally hopeful and optimistic, you'll be less vulnerable. Stress-hardy people tend to embrace challenges, have a stronger sense of humor, believe in a higher purpose, and accept change as an inevitable part of life.

- Your ability to deal with your emotions: If you don't know how to calm and soothe yourself when you're feeling sad, angry, or troubled, you're more likely to become stressed and agitated. Having the ability to identify and deal appropriately with your emotions can increase your tolerance to stress and help you bounce back from adversity.

- Your knowledge and preparation: The more you know about a stressful situation, including how long it will last and what to expect, the easier it is to cope. For example, if you go into surgery with a realistic picture of what to expect post-op, a painful recovery will be less stressful than if you were expecting to bounce back immediately.

Improving Your Ability To Handle Stress

- Get moving: Upping your activity level is one tactic you can employ right now to help relieve stress and start to feel better. Regular exercise can lift your mood and serve as a distraction from worries, allowing you to break out of the cycle of negative thoughts that feed stress. Rhythmic exercises such as walking, running, swimming, and dancing are particularly effective, especially if you exercise mindfully (focusing your attention on the physical sensations you experience as you move).

- Connect to others: The simple act of talking face-to-face with another human can trigger hormones that relieve stress when you're feeling agitated or insecure. Even just a brief exchange of kind words or a friendly look from another human being can help calm and soothe your nervous system. So, spend time with people who improve your mood and don't let your responsibilities keep you from having a social life. If you don't have any close relationships, or your relationships are the source of your stress, make it a priority to build stronger and more satisfying connections.

- Engage your senses Another fast way to relieve stress is by engaging one or more of your senses—sight, sound, taste, smell, touch, or movement. The key is to find the sensory input that works for you. Does listening to an uplifting song make you feel calm? Or smelling ground coffee? Or maybe petting an animal works quickly to make you feel centered? Everyone responds to sensory input a little differently, so experiment to find what works best for you.

- Learn to relax: You can't completely eliminate stress from your life, but you can control how much it affects you. Relaxation techniques such as yoga, meditation, and deep breathing activate the body's relaxation response, a state of restfulness that is the polar opposite of the stress response. When practiced regularly, these activities can reduce your everyday stress levels and boost feelings of joy and serenity. They also increase your ability to stay calm and collected under pressure.

- Eat a healthy diet: The food you eat can improve or worsen your mood and affect your ability to cope with life's stressors. Eating a diet full of processed and convenience food, refined carbohydrates, and sugary snacks can worsen symptoms of stress, while a diet rich in fresh fruit and vegetables, high-quality protein, and omega-3 fatty acids, can help you better cope with life's ups and downs.

- Get your rest: Feeling tired can increase stress by causing you to think irrationally.

At the same time, chronic stress can disrupt your sleep. Whether you're having trouble falling asleep or staying asleep at night, there are plenty of ways to improve your sleep so you feel less stressed and more productive and emotionally balanced.

Chapter 10: Avoiding And Altering The Stressors

Continuing from the previous chapter, we will discuss some simple stress coping strategies that you can use. Shall we get started?

Avoid Unnecessary Stress:

Unsurprisingly, you cannot avoid everything that stresses you out. However, there are those that you can simply cut away from your life without any damage. The thing is, some people tend to attach themselves to these things-- whether it be out of comfort or routine. What can you do?

- Learning how to say no. Create boundaries, be aware of your limit and stick to them. This applies to both your professional and private life. Having too much on your plate at any given time will surely lead to stress, not to mention, people would continue taking advantage of you simply because you let them.

- Avoid the people who cause you stress. If there is someone in your life who consistently causes stress, then reduce the amount of meetings or time you spend with these people. However, if the situation calls for something more drastic, consider ending your relationship with them completely. In some cases, you need to think about yourself first before others.

- Be in control of the environment you are in. You already know the things that can trigger your stress. If something causes you to feel anxious, then avoid it like the plague. If certain topics or conversations make you feel tense, then let the people you are with know about it. They should be understanding enough to avoid speaking of it whenever you're around. Remember, you do not have to deal with something you are uncomfortable with. Always do things in your own time.

- Edit your to-do list well. Look at your schedule and the amount of time you have each day then compare it with your to-do list. Does it remain feasible? Keep in mind that you can drop certain tasks that aren't necessary or even choose to delete them completely.

Altering the Situation:

What happens if you are unable to avoid the stressor? Well, the next logical step is to try and alter it in a way that works for you. There is always a way for you to alter the situation so that it no longer becomes a potential problem. Here are a few simple things you can do to get started with that:

- Learn how to let your feelings out as opposed to bottling them all up. This is something that many people are actually guilty of. Keeping their feelings bottled up instead of communicating them in a more open manner. The thing is, whenever you do this, more and more negative energy begin piling up while the situation remains the same. Change this and be more vocal about your frustrations. It would make a world of difference.

- Accept compromise as an option. It only goes that if you are asking a person to change, then you ought to be willing to apply the same principles to yourself. A bit of compromise can go a long way when it comes to lessening your stress levels.

- Practice assertiveness. When it comes to your life, it is important that you never take a backseat. Being more assertive will allow you to do this as well as lessen the stress you have to deal with. Be more upfront and it will certainly pay off.

- Be better at time management. One of the most common causes of stress is lack of time. However, more often than not, the fault lies in the person himself and not on outside influences. Mismanagement, procrastination or total lack of focus are just some of the reasons why this happens. Try and avoid these issues by prioritizing your tasks and making sure that you have a schedule mapped out for the rest of the day. This results to less frustrations and better productivity.

Chapter 11: Understanding The Sources Of Tension And Stress

The first step to overcoming stress is by identifying and comprehending the sources and reasons of stress in your life. To realize the sources, it is important that you understand that there are two basic types of stress: short-term and long-term. While the former gives you strength under tough situations and motivates you to give your best under pressure, the latter has a destructive effect on your life. It feeds on your health and happiness, making you emotionally crippled with time. This is why it is essential that you find the reasons behind your long-term stress and tackle them.

Identifying the stress triggers

To recognize your stress triggers, you need to sit alone and think about your life in general. Try to find out the time stress just became a part of your life. Once you know that time, you need to further narrow down your research and look for the five or six major events that would have contributed to the mental pressure.

Try to go back in time and think of how you felt in each of those situations. Which event was the most stressful and why? Once you have the answer to this question, you will be aware of the cause of your stress. For instance, it could be your parent's divorce three years back, or it could be the loss of a loved one or the end of a job you loved. Stress can be caused by almost anything that means a lot to you.

Analyze your personality

In addition to doing this, you need to examine your attitude, habits and personality very closely. Most of the time, stress is stimulated because of your behaviors and habits. For instance, some people have a habit of panicking every now and then. Even if nothing is wrong, they feel that things aren't right and something bad is about to happen. This attitude often leads to stress.

Additionally, some people like to blame others for their stress. This is another unhealthy attitude that results in long-term stress. Therefore, by analyzing your personality and attitude, you can get insight into the causes of your stress. Once you know all the major stress triggers in your life, you need to list them down, so you can practice the second step.

Manage Stress Triggers Under Your Control

The second step to managing your stress involves considering the things that you can control on your own. The causes of stress can be broadly divided into two categories: things you did wrong and things that others around you are doing wrong. While you can rectify your mistakes, you cannot coerce somebody to behave in a certain manner. If they don't understand that they are at fault, you cannot change their perspective.

However, most victims of stress aren't able to realize this, which is why they are never successful in regulating and alleviating their stress. If you want to live a calm and peaceful life, then you need to differentiate between the stress caused by your own issues and that caused by others. For that, you need to use the list of stress triggers you made in the first step.

Finding out what stress triggers you can control

Take your list that has all your stress triggers and think about each trigger for a couple of minutes to realize whether it is caused by your own behavior and you can control it. Once you have analyzed your list, you need to sort out the triggers into two categories: ones you can control and others that aren't in your control. Next, you need to understand how you can deal with the different triggers and which ones you need to let go off.

For instance, if your lack of confidence makes you stressful in situations where you need to speak in front of people, then it is something you can control. You need to muster up courage and battle your demons for being able to speak in public and mitigate your stress pertinent to this fear. Similarly, find out all the stress triggers that are controllable, so you can manage them using different techniques that will be discussed in the following chapters.

Letting go of things not in your control

On the other hand, if your colleague's rude and unsupportive behavior freaks you out, then this is something out of your reach. You cannot control their behavior. If they cannot fathom what their behavior is doing to you, then there is nothing you can do to change their behavior. However, you can do something that will help you deal with this. You can make your mind realize and understand the fact that, your colleague will continue to behave in a certain manner, but you need to change your perspective. You need to live your life your way without giving them any importance.

Not paying heed to the stress caused by others is tough, but once you understand that you aren't responsible for it, you can mitigate it with the aid of helpful techniques and practices.

Chapter 12: Visualize Your Future

What if you woke up in the morning and just made the decision that you can have whatever you wanted? It was already finalized. A done deal. What if you admitted that your dreams are in fact or reality? That they are there for a reason. That if you just start fighting for them. They would manifest into reality. How would you feel?

If you could trade in worrying about everything and start celebrating, how would you feel? If you could do everything you wanted to do and have everything you wanted and simply just enjoy life.

Here's the thing. All that is possible and it's possible for you. It's not just dreams for other people. You qualify as well. Here's the problem. You haven't done anything to make this a reality. You haven't asked for it or assumed that it would be yours and acted as if it was already. Most likely you don't believe that it's realistic for that. Maybe you don't think you deserve it, but spending your life stressing over your situation isn't helping either.

So what if you got to lose? If you were to instead dream about what you want and then act as if you already have it, still better than what you're doing now. Because what you're doing now isn't working. You're allowing stress to consume you and that isn't doing anything to change your situation.

I will tell you that if you don't do something different, nothing will ever change for you. If you're not about your dreams, then you won't achieve them. You'll never see them manifest into reality. If you don't do something different and walked toward it and allow stress to grow and fester, you're looking at a life of depression and health problems.

Get out there and do something about it. Take massive action right now. How you talk to yourself and how you phrase things in your mind makes all the difference. Mindset is key to achieving your dreams and turning them into realities. When you speak in such a way that you convince yourself that you've already achieved these things, it programs your mind to start making those statements a reality. Your mind is an incredibly powerful thing, but we have to know how to use it the right way.

In order for it to work for us. You have to claim those things that you want and you have to act as if you already have them. That's all there is to it. That's when the stress starts alleviating in your life and good things are to happen. But this only happens if you don't give up. It's your responsibility to keep going on, to keep pushing yourself to keep trying. Just one more time. It's always just one more time.

Be the person that you always wanted to be and that others see in you. There are people waiting to be inspired by you. There are people waiting for your help, but they need you to be who you were meant to be. You're the only one who can take action to make things happen in your life every single day. You're the only one who can reach out and get exactly what you want. Nobody's going to do it for you. You need to accept nothing less then the best for yourself. Ask yourself to constantly what you want and then own it because it's already yours. Believing in yourself is all it takes to make that decision and then taking action on that decision is what gets you exactly what you want.

Do the Work

Stress management can be complicated. It's just a matter of doing the work necessary to manage it every single day, week after week and being consistent. So when someone is complaining that they are too stressed out and they can't "adult" today, I really can't even deal with it. I can't go there. I can't respond genuinely and look them in the eyes because it's a bunch of crap. You're just not being patient.

Patience is something that we all need to learn in this day and age when everything is instant gratification. Patience is becoming an endangered species, but the one thing that separates those who live a stress free life from those who don't is patience.

It's the internal dialogue and how you train your brain that determines your stress level. There are always going to be things that test your patience and frustrate you. It takes time to learn stress management techniques. You can't read one book and then assume that your life is going to improve. Not without doing the work every day. You have to implement the techniques and it has to be reinforced constantly.

You will find there are things in your life every day that will trigger you to feel stressed out. You have to immediately change your state of mind into one that is peaceful, calling, and patient. But if that's too much work for you then you need to accept the fact that you will always be a stressed out individual.

Nothing is going to work for you because you're not willing to put in the work. Not everyone can live a calm, stress-free life because they choose to get stressed out about things they have no control over. In fact, it can become an addiction. It can become a habit so strong that their immediate reaction is to stress out. And then the body's physical reaction matches the emotional, mental reaction, it can cause problems.

The good news is that you can change this around 180° to condition your body not to react physically to stressful situations. But again, it takes time. Are you willing to put in the time? Are you willing to be patient? Are you willing to take the effort required and apply it to changing your life you can have a peaceful life? Do what you have to do in order to get this resolved. Hire a counselor. Work with a coach.

Have someone hold you accountable to journal daily. Do research about the right types of methodologies and tips that will allow you to minimize stress. Do more of what you love to do. Whether that's writing. Her hobbies are crafts, and most importantly, be consistent every single day. You have to persevere. Nothing will change much more willing to meet it at the finish line and be willing to go beyond if necessary.

Chapter 13: The Effects Of Stress On The Mind

The effects that stress has on the human mind can be very negative. The health of the human mind is so in tune with your emotions that every stressful situation that it encounters will have a lasting effect on the mind. This is also evident when the build-up of stressful situations becomes too much for the human mind to control. Stress can have so many negative effects on the human mind that people that deal with high stress situations regularly are more prone to many mental illnesses. Stress can actually make your mind even more susceptible to illnesses such as depression, anxiety, Post Traumatic Stress Disorder, panic attacks, and many more. Post Traumatic Stress Disorder is one of the most debilitating mental illnesses that can be caused by an abundance of stress alone. PTSD patients don't react to stress the way that the average person does.

Their trauma has essentially destroyed the person's "fight or flight" response, and they no longer react to stress in the most natural way that a person can. Instead the stress they feel can come at random moments, and they can't suppress the feeling. It is common for PTSD patients to exhibit signs of high stress in times where they should not be feeling any signs of stress at all. This inability to use the mind's natural "fight or flight" response to stress causes severe mood swings, emotional flashbacks, night terrors, disturbing thoughts, and more. It is also very common for people that suffer from PTSD to become emotionally withdrawn, and suffer from severe depression.

Post Traumatic Stress Disorder is not the only mental illness that is created or made worse through stress. Stress has numerous effects on a lot of different diseases of the mind. Manic depression, severe anxiety, and even dementia can be dramatically affected by the abundance of stress. Stress makes these mental disorders much harder to deal with, and can cause them to worsen quickly. It is important to remember the ways that stress can cause current health concerns to worsen, and to try to eliminate certain stressors that become long term triggers. Doing so will help you deal with mental illness without having your treatment plan disrupted by stressful situations. Stress affects people with mental illnesses much more strongly.

Some of the effects that stress has on the mind can be dealt with a little more easily than a severe mental illness. At the very least, prolonged exposure to stressors in life can lead to aggression or depression. Lashing out at others for little reason, or becoming more withdrawn from friends and family are two less serious ways that stress can affect the mind. Although it is no small thing to be feeling depressed, typical depression is easier to deal with than a more serious stress related mental illness. Stress is known to make people feel fatigued for little reason, other than the mind can shut down the production of insulin during times of high stress.

The human mind is a very intricate and fragile organ. It is responsible for creating the sensation of stress, but it can also be hurt by the sensation of stress. In a sense, the human mind is only hurting itself. The mind can also use stress to its advantage. Some athletes are said to be "clutch" performers. Really, that just means that they perform best under high stress situations. The same can be said for anyone. You don't have to be a world class athlete to use stress to your advantage. People from all sorts of jobs can use stress in a positive fashion. Cooks, stock brokers, doctors, construction workers, and even fast food employees all have very stressful jobs. Some people may excel in that type of environment, and use the stress of the job to help them do better.

Using stress as an advantage does have its own risks, however. Just because stress is being used to help someone perform better, doesn't mean that it won't have a negative long term impact on that person. The result of several hundred small situations may result in a lot of damage to the mind of an individual, even if they honestly believe that they are using stress to their advantage. Stress is still stress, and in the long run it can have very negative impact on the human mind. It may not feel like you are doing yourself an injustice if you are thriving in a high stress lifestyle, but you could still be doing just as much damage to your brain as anyone. Stress has an impact on the brain, where over time, the impact cannot be reversed.

Stress has also been found to actually damage the human brain physically, over time. A Yale University report, published in the journal "Biological Psychiatry", found that stressful life events could shrink parts of the human brain. The report also found that this shrinkage in the brain could make it harder for people to regulate their emotions, and even their metabolism. In other words, stress can physically affect your brain in a way that it will lead to even more stress, in the future. And also, it is harder to maintain a healthy body after dealing with stressful events. The way the shrinkage affects metabolism can make your body have a more difficult time breaking down proteins and amino acids to create healthy energy. Also, the affects of the shrinkage of the brain will make your body have a more difficult time maintaining healthy glucose and insulin levels.

People suffering from underlying mental illnesses are more susceptible to the adverse affects of stress. Diseases like dementia, Alzheimer's disease, schizophrenia, and bipolar disorder are known to become worse or flare up when stressful situations are more abundant. The reason why stress affects people with mental illness more adversely isn't necessarily concrete, but most scientists agree that suffering from mental illness makes people more susceptible to the adverse affects of stress because the mind is already in a weakened state. Having a mental illness may make it extremely difficult to deal with high stress situations.

The way that stress affects the mind is going to depend on a case by case situation. Everybody has different perceptions of stressful events, and so dealing with the problem is going to be different for everyone. The best way to interpret your own needs when dealing with stress is to understand how it is affecting your own mind. How do you react to stress? Do you exhibit signs of the "fight or flight" response? Or, does stress affect your mind in a more extreme way? These questions are some of the most important that you will have to answer, in order to reverse the damage that stress can do to your mind. Evaluate the stressor that you deal with on a daily basis, and figure out ways to help you cope with them more safely.

Stress affects the mind in more ways than are currently known, so there is no sure way to understand the full affects that stress causes. Some people and a negative can view stress as a positive by others, but the fact is that can have life altering affects on some people. Take heed of what your body and mind are trying to tell you, because sometimes that is the best way to understand how stress affects you directly. Even if you aren't suffering from a mental illness caused by stress, it is good to recognize the signs of too much stress on the mind.

Chapter 14: What Are The Stages Of Stress Management?

Before we encroach into the subject of steps of stress management, let's first familiarize ourselves with what Stress Management is. Stress, as we discussed in chapter one, is nothing but a mental pressure. The ways in which we deal with stress are together called Stress Management. It means not to prevent it. That would be Stress Prevention.

Stress Management, on the other hand, is a step that has to be taken after stress has set in. It is a damage control mode of action. The various ways in which we tackle the invasion of stress into our mental realm consist of the methods of stress management. Remember it is about management, which means there is little prevention and more dealing involved.

Stress Management is divided into three primary stages. They are discussed below along with some helpful illustrations to go with them. Let's start our journey:

Stage I – Recognition

It is of supreme importance that you are able to identify what exactly is causing you stress. The source of your stress is where all the solutions lie. It is only when you find the root that you can uproot the tree or kill it slowly but surely.

The importance of this stage can be grasped from the following points:

The very fact that you are aware of the source of your worries is half the job done. It is only by knowledge that we stand to get into the battle stage of the treatment.

When you know the source, therein lays the answer too. It so happens that the source is often also the provider of the key to an issue. Instead of looking answers elsewhere, focus all your attention on the source.

The origin of your stress speaks a lot about what sort of things cause stress in your life. When you have identified the origin, similar troubles in the future could be easily avoided by recognizing the pattern in which stress affects you.

For example, someone is stressed about his car breaking down. Now it may have been due to his inherent quality to get attached to things. Or it could also may have been because the car is a helpful factor in him reaching his office where sits a boss who calls the shots; yes including the one where he shouts at employees for reaching office late. Here, you will be addressing two sources of stresses in your life by identifying one.

Stage one is thereby, a passage to further keys to other sources. It is not a simple and single step; it's a continuation of sorts.

Stage II – Elimination

It's easier said than done. You can go about the process of eliminating your stress in various ways. You could either totally ignore it or you could solve it. The latter suggestion works better than the former one but that's not always the case. When you ignore an issue, it breeds and gets multiplied in terms of intensity.

It stays neglected, only to pop up in future with many more heads, like a scary demon. So it's generally safe to solve a stress than ignore it. However, some stresses are better ignored since they are issues that have no promise of getting solved; you'll only be wasting your time and energy on trying to work it out.

So, the primary question remains; how to go about eliminating the stress? Here are some tips to carry out under this stage:

·Now that you have successfully identified the stress source, try to kill it. If that's not possible or is proving to be more work than it deserves, try lessening its symptoms.

·Elimination is best performed when you are in high spirits. Develop a positive attitude towards life and embark on the journey of elimination.

·Believe in yourself. It is vital that you have the self-belief to carry out elimination. Killing a stress is not easy. Sometimes, we are so attached with the stress that we warm up to it. A dear relative might be a stress but due to your proximity, you refuse to sort it out. Avoid such thinking as it proves disadvantageous for you in the end.

·Be confident enough to start the process of elimination. When you decide to eliminate a problem from your life, you must be bubbling with self-confidence. Simply believing in your own self won't work; you also have to show self-confidence.

Equip yourself with the requisite mental strength to go through the stages.

Elimination is the stage when you solve the issue and not further complicate it. Many people have this stage backfiring on themselves because they mess up the entire process. Bring clarity inside your head regarding how you are going to do it.

You could complete the process by talking, performing, body language, writing or even a mere application of mind. Do not be of two minds. If you have decided on a course, do not deviate from it.

Stage III – Prevention

Now that you have successfully eliminated the stress from your life, it is time for preventing further stress from entering your life in the future. You are now familiar with how it feels to taste a sigh of relief after stress is eradicated from your life. You are content knowing that you no longer have to spend hours worrying and brooding over a single issue.

You are aware that your time and energy can now be spent on matters that really deserve your attention and attendance. You can prevent future stress by simply devoting your focus to things that you had missed out on while wasting time stressing yourself out.

These are some of the ticks to help you with completely preventing stress from further entering your life:

·Do not go running back to past stresses. Once a thing is done, it should be forgotten. There is no point trying to get into a mess you got out of.

·Harden yourself according to trying situations. It is only when you fall weak, emotionally and otherwise, that you fall prey to stress. Make a priority list of things that matter to you. Make another list of things that don't. Compare the two lists and make sure you fill up the latter with as much things as you can.

·Guard against being easy. The most common cause of stress is ease. It's when people become easily available and vulnerable that they invite stressful situations. When you can be easily talked to, everyone takes you for granted. People do not value you as much as they value someone who keeps a distance from easy company. Of course, I do not imply that you become unsocial all of a sudden. However, being picky about your friendships and groups wouldn't hurt. You will come out as an independent, classy and a very particular individual.

This stage aims at making refining you as a person who isn't vulnerable to possibilities of stress. Not everyone is mentally strong enough to ward of stress when it comes knocking at the door. This stage will surely show a stark difference between those who can and those who cannot. Regardless, you have to show some spirit and take up the challenge. It is important that you shed off your old skin and start creating a new shining one. This new skin will not only keep you protected from stress but will also develop your personality to extreme levels.

Chapter 15: Defining Success

"Success is not the key to happiness. Happiness is the key to success. If you love what you are doing you will be successful." Albert Schweitzer

Success consists of far more than the sum of our material goods. It is an intangible thing that people can only define for themselves. It is that elusive intangibility that seems to have created more confusion around this subject than anything else. The world hates intangibles and prefers to offer clear-cut examples, and so, with little more definite to work with, it has presented the acquisition of wealth or power as its most obvious representation of success. Rich business executives, powerful politicians and famous celebrities are the people who are most likely to be presented as role models in our distorted society. While wealth and power are seen as desirable we need to recognize that those are not the only factors by which success should be rated. Failure to broaden that definition leads to a distorted society in which we cease to have regard for the important services provided by the likes of nurses, artists, social workers and others whose valuable input so often goes unrecognized; a world where those people doing the thousands of comparatively mundane day to day tasks that keep our society functioning are disregarded or even perceived as 'losers'.

We have become so mesmerized by these distorted versions of success that we even pass them on to our children as we encourage them to go down paths toward financially lucrative careers with little regard to where their true talents or yearnings may lie. It is now estimated that more than fifty percent of American's are unhappy in their jobs and yet instead of teaching our children to root out their passions we persist in advancing the idea that the acquisition of wealth is the true path to success.

The popular consensus seems to be that we must work hard which will lead to success that in turn will lead to happiness. As psychologists and science research the subject in greater depth we are beginning to see that the popular consensus has got the equation the wrong way around and that people who intentionally follow a course toward happiness tend to work harder and become more successful as a result.

This is not to promote the idea that wealth is necessarily a bad thing or that poverty is in any way to be admired as an alternative. The idea is that we should each choose our own version of what we feel represents success to us rather than simply accepting the example that most of the modern world seems so intent on promoting. Success is subjective and it needs to remain that way if we are to really reach our full potentials rather than just accept a one size fits all route to fulfillment.

One of the many dictionary definitions of success is: The accomplishment of an aim or purpose. It is a short little definition which somewhat understates the immensity of the task. To accomplish an aim or purpose is one thing but what if you are not sure what that aim or purpose should be. Far too many of us fail to wrestle with this subject and instead we simply accept the prevailing view that pursuit of material gains or recognition by our peers is what success is all about. Is it any wonder that so many of us are unhappy in our jobs, feel unfulfilled or suffer from a deep sense of failure when these objectives are not achieved?

Each of us needs to set our own definition of success and then to own it. On the road toward success this is probably the hardest obstacle to cross. It takes time and a deep examination of what our personal values and desires really are. As your life evolves so your desires and values may evolve too and it is likely that you will have to do an in depth inventory of where you are going at various stages of your life. Your definition of success on leaving college may change by the time you have children or when you decide to retire. Those changes are not to be feared as long as you analyze them honestly and don't allow yourself to be battered by the prevailing views of the world about you or what your peers will think of your decision. It does not matter if the vision you come up with for your own personal success is that of a highly influential businessperson or creative artist. What does matter is that you generate a vision of yourself as successful no matter what field of endeavor you might choose. In many ways these are going to be some of the most important decisions of your life, and while the remainder of this book will try to help you implement those decisions, the actual definition of your version of success has to come from you.

The key to success in any project or venture is to visualize yourself in that position to begin with and then you have something concrete to work towards. Take mental note of the thoughts that pass through your mind throughout each day. Are these thoughts about success and happiness and remaining positive or are they about failure and disappoint and unhappiness? Your frame of mind is often the deciding factor between obtaining success or going up in a hail of flames.

You must always remember that your physical world is a reflection of what is going on in your mental world. If all you thing about are doom, gloom and failure then there is no possible way that you could outwardly reflect anything other than that.

The stronger your positive mental images and thoughts, the more chance that your physical world will portray positive notes and attract positive energies.

Your inner thoughts and emotions are the eyes through which you view the world and how you see certain situations. These thoughts and emotions are also the meter by which your reactions towards a situation are measured and influence your actions and reactions. If you always visualize and think about failure and unhappiness, you will never be able to see the possible silver lining in a situation and your reactions will not encourage that silver lining but rather the worst possible outcome.

Every person is different in the emotions, thought patterns and behavior and every person has a focus on different thoughts. For this reason, no one person's reaction to situations or events will ever be a mirror image of those of another person. One person may perhaps have insecurities about themselves and think that they are not deserving of recognition, this will cause them to outwardly reflect these thoughts by not bestowing recognition on another who may deserve it. In doing so they are creating a negative situation which is centered around what they think are their own shortcomings. Another may realize that they have flaws but rather than focus on these flaws, the will focus on their positive and strong points and this may come across as confidence and allow them to be self-assured. They may be confident enough to pass recognition on to others who are deserving. If you follow the positive traits of the latter, you are guaranteed to begin to attract recognition of your own.

Creative visualization is a visualization technique in which you focus all your mental thoughts and energy on a positive outcome to an event or situation and you visualize that event or situation in a positive manner. This technique of visualizing success and happiness is what tends to draw those things ever closer. Everybody possesses the ability to use creative visualization we are just not aware that we are using it unconsciously and are therefore not focusing and directing it in a positive manner.

Your mind is your own best friend or worst enemy. Train your mind and yourself to reach that goal of success and happiness.

Become conscious of the power you hold within yourself to reach your goals and stop thinking negatively. Negativity is a breeding ground for more negativity.

You need to portray certain traits and put these into action on a daily basis in order to achieve success and the resulting happiness. You need to first have faith in yourself and your abilities. If you believe in yourself, you give others reason to believe too. Patience is key to any process, we must remember that all things that really are worthwhile do not happen overnight and take hard work so be patient and you will reach your goal. Perseverance is an amazing trait that shows your ability to rise above your mistakes and misgivings and take another shot. You will never achieve success if you give up after failing one time. Concentration and willpower work hand in hand. To begin with it is going to take a lot of concentration and mental power to consciously focus your mental thoughts in a positive manner. You have to train yourself and your mind to think in a particular way, which it is unaccustomed to. You will need the strength of your willpower to stop yourself from falling back into the same old routine and thought patterns that bred negativity in the past. Discipline yourself to keep reverting back to positive thoughts and energy should your mind begin to wander back to the dark side. Self-discipline is possibly the most difficult thing to achieve. To achieve success in anything, you need to have the ambition and drive to reach that success. If you have ambition you will be willing to do whatever it takes to get to where you want to be.

We must keep in mind that success in so only the result of what we are doing but also of how we are doing. The act of performing the duties is important but so is the state of mind while doing it. Doing the hard work is important but it is not the only thing that matters during this process. Sometimes we become so wrapped up in the actual goal that we are trying to achieve that we forget about the joy our work should bring us. If there is no joy during the process or enjoyment while doing the task, then the task is not worth doing. It becomes monotonous and boring and you will not give it your best attention. The outcome or result with then obviously be affected.

Let go of habits that keep you in a negative frame of mind and adopt habits that promote the positive, happiness you wish to achieve. Pursue your own natural talents and abilities and pursue work you enjoy and have a passion for. Stop trying to change who you are to please others or to obtain the approval of others. Love yourself and be happy with the choices you make for you are the only one who has to live with those choices.

Be true to yourself, live by your own code and have the courage to voice your opinions and thoughts. Believe in yourself and your worth and others will follow suit. Confidence that radiates from within, shines brightly allowing others to feel your confidence and will start to believe in your opinions and your ideas and put their support behind you.

Believe that success is already yours for your thoughts are the seeds of what the outcome will be. The power is yours, you just need to learn how to harness it. Take control of your own future, happiness and success.

Chapter 16: Other Effective Methods

There are other simple but powerful techniques you can use to fight stress that can't easily fit into the categories that we have just seen. However, don't underestimate them. These techniques are worth their weight in gold. Here are a few of them:

20: Set Aside Some "Me-Time"

There is a saying "All work and no play make Jack a dull boy."

This is truer today than ever. The modern life today dictates that you work, work, and then work some more. The problem is; this paradigm is bad for your body. You need some time off for your body to reset. You need some time to truly enjoy the activities you value outside work.

This isn't me giving you general information by the way: WebMD reports taking time off for hobbies as one of the top ways to manage stress. Watch a movie, play golf, take the kids to the park, go swimming...Do whatever pleases you out of work.

They even go on to say that you do not have to invest too much time. 15 to 20 minutes a day sometimes just seems to do the trick. But if I were you, I'd dedicate more time than that.

21: Get Enough Exercise

Yet another way you may reduce your stress is by getting plenty of exercise.

The Mayo Clinic reports that any form of exercise is a natural antidote to stress. This is good because you do not have to come up with a complicated workout regime for you to be effective. One Hollywood Real Estate broker I know who works long hours, 7 days a week, jogs every morning before he starts his day and he says this helps him relieve his pressure.

But why is exercise good for managing stress?

It's actually simple.

For one thing, exercise produces hormones known as endorphins. Endorphins are your body's natural "feel good" chemicals. The Anxiety and Depression Association of America calls them natural painkillers that help counter the effects of stress. They also help you get better sleep and this helps with your overall stress problem.

So, starting today, you can start creating some time for exercise. You do not even have to exercise for long like the gym goers.

You do not even need to go to the gym or even buy gym equipment at all. I work out every day for 30 minutes in my house. I only do squats, pushups, crunches and sit-ups. I am fit and I rarely get stressed. You can do the same.

22: Study Some History

It may sound absurd for you to realize that by reading some history, you could fight some of the stress that you currently have?

But how? Let me explain...

The truth is; one of the reasons why most people are stressed is because many people fear what the future brings. The APA reports that two thirds of Americans stress out because of the future.

If you are anxious about the future, you should simply go to the library and take a history book. It doesn't matter which one; just pick any.

By studying a little bit of history, you will realize that the world is always becoming a better place. The world that you live in right now is infinitely better than the world that existed even just a decade ago.

This trend should help you get things in proper focus. Things are always getting better, not worse. You should relax and welcome the future instead.

23: Live One Day At A Time

Another secret to fighting stress is living one day at a time.

The thing is; you usually cannot tackle all your life problems in one day. Furthermore, there is never a life without problems. Problems are always coming up every time. I learnt this after reading Mark Manson's **"The Art of not giving a F***k."**

In the book, he paints a picture of how our expectation of a life without problems is unrealistic and tends to cause anxiety and dissatisfaction.

What you can do in order to maintain peace of mind is to take on things, one day at a time. Forget the past that is already gone. Let go of trying to imagine what will happen in the future. Today is your only certainty.

Concentrate on doing everything that you can do today. Let go of everything else. In other words, live your life just until you go to bed. You will find that most of your stress goes away when you do just that.

24: Share Your Troubles With Others

One of the reasons why stress is so prevalent in society is because people like to keep things to themselves.

However, it may come as a surprise to you to realize that sharing your problems with someone can help reduce your stress. This is according to a study by Marshall School of Business titled "Two stressed people equals less stress".

The study revealed that this technique works well especially if you talk to someone who understands your position or has been through a similar situation or is even going through it.

So, you may benefit from this technique by finding someone who you are close with and who you trust. Then you can always talk to that person from time to time, when you feel encumbered by stress. You will find that doing so helps lift the off weight from you and you feel better.

If you do not have many people who are supportive in your life, you can look for support groups online. For instance, Alcoholics Anonymous is a famous example. There are many others that are on social media. Others are offline. This link can help you identify some good ones.

25: Talk To A Professional Counselor

Finally, you also have the option of talking to a professional counselor.

Even though much of what we have discussed works very well, there are certain stress levels and situations that may need the intervention of a certified professional.

For instance, your stress may be as a result of a major trauma you suffered in the past. Or there could be a deep underlying problem in your subconscious that is preventing you from effectively combating your stress.

Those are things that only a professional can deal with. A professional may even prescribe medication that may help you get through your problem easily.

So, if you have tried everything that we have just discussed and your problem seems to persist, that may be a sure sign that you need professional help.

Fortunately, finding professional help isn't difficult. Walk into any major health center and you are likely to find Psychologists as well as Psychiatrists working there. When you do find them, do not hesitate to ask for their services.

Chapter 17: Stress Relief And Spirituality

Some stress relief tools Are Substantial Eating foods that are healthy and speaking with friends. A method is by way of spirituality."Taking the path less traveled by researching your Spirituality may result in a better life goal, better personal connections, and improved stress control..." -- Mayo Clinic team"Adopting the Ideal attitude can convert a negative stress into a favorable one." -- Dr. Hans SelyeStress has developed a terrible reputation. High-stress amounts during a long period have been implicated in increased risk for several ailments, including hypertension, cardiovascular disease, asthma, reduced resistance, obesity, diabetes, cancer, infections, inflammations, headaches, digestive issues, and aging. Stress, depression, and substance abuse Also have been demonstrated to be stress-related. So it appears that we do cover a price. When we look, we discover that not all stress is bad. Stress can be harmful, right, or neutral. When we look much closer, we find that we can make decisions that may significantly decrease the negative effect of Stress and, at times, even turn trying challenges to positive growth-filled experiences. Stress is inside people and both out people. Stress is the Outer “stuff" that occurs. The concern involves all the changes that occur in our own lives, the demands all that we encounter, and each of the challenges we confront. Fear is inside people. The experience of stress comes in how we view and how we react to problems, demands, and the modifications in our own lives. The strain experience is the mix of our ideas, feelings, and biological reactions to the outside “stuff" that occurs. One individual can run a long-distance at a steady speed from fear. The other individual can run an identical interval at a fast pace. Every person's experience is different, although the action might be comparable. For the Individual motivated by panic, Long run conduct is made even harder from the subjective experience of distress (negative stress). In the light of their knowledge of faith and hope, the strain of this conduct fades for the individual driven by a dream.Dr. Hans Seyle is popularly called the" Father of Modern Stress Research." The design started his lifelong investigations to the effect of stress, and he reasoned it is likely to have Stress without distress -- fear without consequences. The right is being proven by research, and spirituality can be an instrument by which we can turn potentially harmful stress to an encounter. Studies have been revealing that meditation and prayer enhance the health and wellness dangers related to Stress. Meditation was linked to a decreased risk of cardiovascular disease, lower blood stress, stress, and risk for diabetes. Participation at a community was proven to be associated with life span, enhanced function aging, and Stress. Does spirituality lower the effect of Stress? Do challenges that are stressful alter? By altering the significance we give to these 19, the results of events can alter. Our practices developing how we view problems, and trust -- can help keep us grounded in our values; religion reduces distress' experience.

When stress is meditation, prayer and continuing may disrupt chronic stress' expertise with minutes of renewal and serenity. Tension with periods of renewal reduces the health risks credited to Stress. Since our spirituality helps us feel part of something larger spirituality can alter the experience of stress. When we align with a Higher Power, we are inclined to feel helpless in the face of the challenges of life. In a manner, belonging to a religious or religious community can decrease the feeling of being weak in the front of migraines that are major and alone. It's well recognized that a community's aid elicits the effects of Stress. It is a fantastic idea to keep on eating a Nutritious Diet. It's equally a great idea to utilize our practice to decrease the effect of stress.

The planet can start to feel like a place once we allow ourselves to feel part of something larger than ourselves. Finding significance and beliefs make chances for mastery and can lessen distress. The negative side of Stress faded when it interrupted with all the minutes of peace, is softened by the community, and seasoned through the energy of religion.

What's Spirituality?

Spirituality has many definitions, but in its heart Spirituality will help to give your life circumstances. It is not attached to spiritual worship or a belief system. It originates from the relationship with yourself and with the evolution of your value system, others, along with your look for meaning in life. For most requires the Kind of spiritual Observance, prayer, meditation, or even a belief in a higher power. For many others, it may be discovered in a geographical area, music, artwork, or nature. Spirituality differs for everybody.

How Does Spirituality Help With Stress Relief?

It has many benefits for stress relief and general Psychological wellness. It can assist you

Feel a sense of purpose. Cultivating your spirituality can Help discover what is most meaningful in your lifetime. You remove Stress and can concentrate less.

Connect to the entire world. The more you believe that you have a purpose. If you are alone, the solitary, you will feel -- even. This may result in peace that is valuable during tough times.

Release control. When you are feeling a part of a greater whole, May, understand that you are not accountable. It's possible to share the joys of life's blessings in addition to a load of times.

Expand your service network. Whether you find on character walks with a buddy, or in your loved ones, At a church, mosque or synagogue, this sharing of expression helps build relationships.

Lead a more healthy life. Individuals who believe themselves Spiritual might encounter health benefits and may be able to deal with Stress.

Finding Your Spirituality

Some self-discovery may be taken by uncovering your spirituality. Here are some questions to ask to find out what values and experiences specify you:

What are your significant relationships?

What do you appreciate most in your lifetime?

You are given a feeling of community by what people?

What gives you expect and motivates you?

What brings you joy?

Which are your proudest accomplishments?

The answers to these questions can help you identify the maximum Individuals and adventures in your lifetime. You can concentrate your search for spirituality on actions and the connections in life. Who has helped identify you as Personal individual development?

Cultivating Your Spirituality

Spirituality entails getting in touch self. There is an element of self-reflection. **Try these hints:**

Try mindfulness, meditation, prayer, and relaxation methods to help focus your ideas and find peace of mind.

Keep a journal that will assist you in documenting your progress and expressing your emotions.

Look for a trusted adviser. Others might have insights you have found.

Read essays or stories that will assist you in evaluating unique aspects of life.

Speak. Ask questions to find out how they found their way into a life that is fulfilling.

Nurturing Your Relationships

Your relationships with others nurture spirituality. It's vital to cultivate relationships. **This may result in the sense of the place in life and at the good.**

Make relationships with family a priority and friends. Give more than you get.

See the good in yourself and people. Accept others as they are.

Contribute to a community.

Pursuing A Religious Life

Staying connected with the lifestyles and your soul of those about you can improve your wellbeing, both physically and emotionally. Your notion of spirituality can affect your age and lifestyle experiences, but it continually creates the cornerstone of your well-being, makes it possible to deal with migraines big and small, and also supports your purpose in your life.

Four Religious Strategies To Decrease Stress

Listed below are some for doing this, Hints.

Meditate frequently. I've been meditating for many years, and I'm convinced it is the trick to all our ills. How can this reduce Stress? By allowing us the room to sit down silently in God's existence, concentrate on the breathing or even a word/phrase, and watch and give up our ideas. Anything we focus on, whatever we do not focus on, and raises, reduces. We center on confidence, God, peacefulness, willingness, and also the second. We let go of stress and ideas, the ago that is imperfect, along with the potential. We create room for perfection and the peace of the Holy Spirit to emerge. Get out in nature daily. How is a religious proposal, you may ask. My response infused with intellect and grace? Each time that I connect with life in the tiniest way, I think love and its healing, and my Stress flows from me. My 13-year-old granddaughter Taylor commented after coming out of a chilly walk to and from the library, "That felt great. It had been so calm looking in the blue skies and trees" It is great when we, for example, Taylor, can have a stroll or play tennis outside or something comparable. But even when we cannot, we could all step out at night and look at the moon, take some deep breaths as we walk into our car in the early hours, or see and be thankful for the natural universe as we're driving.

Build your confidence in God. Here is the antidote to stress/fear. You can construct this hope by reading motivational books, replicating supporting biblical passages, discovering and being thankful for all God's blessings, or even listening to music. I highly recommend a CD called Come, Holy Mother, by Kathryn Christian. It includes incredible songs, according to themes of confidence in God from afar as well as mystics. Whenever I hear them or sing together (which I frequently do), I believe God was saying, "Carol, I'm with you. Calm down. All is well."Simplify your lifetime. One of my principles in purchasing something or carrying on something brand new is, "Can this life?" If this is so, I don't do it. Dispossessing yourself of substance possessions/activities is undoubtedly a spiritual practice advocated by scripture. Jesus had small and lived peacefully and joyfully in God. And we could do precisely the same.

Chapter 18: Stress In Your Workplace

You can admit it—even though you enjoy what you're doing, sometimes you feel that your job, your boss, and your work place are the things that are the main sources of your stress. In fact, there are times when you believe that quitting your job or looking for another career is the answer to free yourself from pressure. You don't have to feel guilty when you think or feel these things because you are not alone. In fact, surveys administered in the United States say that 40% of employees view their jobs as the main stressor in their lives, while 30% feel that they are often "burned out" or stressed because of their work; the remaining 30% believe that their health problems are associated with their work-related stress. In the UK, 500,000 workers believe that their stress at work is making them ill and five million individuals in the UK admitted that they are extremely stressed at work.

To add to that, health experts believe that employees are facing a greater threat in their health because of job-related stress now compared to the previous decades. Doctors deem that stress at work could put someone at risk of harmful physical and emotional problems, especially when the requirements of the job exceed the capabilities or the resources of the employee.

Causes of Work-Related Stress

There are a lot of factors that can cause stress at work, and it also depends on the characteristics of the workers, whether they see a factor as a stressor or not. Some of the major causes of work-related stress according to research are: **work overload**, where one is required to work long hours and meet unrealistic deadlines; **management style,** or when employees feel that they lack freedom in their job (everything has to be approved by the management); **work relationships**, where there is poor communication between co-workers and managers; **no work-life**

balance, or when work is already interfering with a worker's personal life; and **salary and benefits**.

Effects of Work-Related Stress

Whether you can relate to one, two, or all of the causes I listed above, the bottom line is that stress at work is inevitable. Even if you look for another job, stress will always be present. The only thing that you have to do is to learn how to cope with it. Why? That's because stress hinders your productivity and directly affects your performance at work. Whenever you're pressured, your creativity and problem-solving skills are limited. Other than that, stress, even if it's acute could cause health problems such as headache, stomach pains, and difficulty sleeping. Chronic stress could lead to even more dangerous complications such as insomnia, hypertension, and anxiety.

Ways to Control Work-Related Stress

Like I mentioned, it's impossible for you to avoid stress entirely, especially at work.

However, in order to avoid the adverse effects of it, what you need to do is learn how to manage it. Here are some ways for you to cope with work-related stress:

Balance Your Schedule

You are only human. Dedicating 24/7 to work will only burn you out and cause stress. What you need to do is create balance in your life. You work to live but you don't live to work, so give yourself time to live your life! Assess your responsibilities and your tasks at work; create a schedule that will let you work and play. Find balance between your career, your family life, and your social life. Stop wishful thinking; take that next plane out to your dream vacation whenever you can.

Beat Procrastination

Why do you dread deadlines even if your boss gave you enough time to work on your report? Well, you probably didn't start working on the project right away! You kept on letting your task sit on your desk for a long time before realizing that you only have a few days left to finish the job you were supposed to do. So what's the solution to beat procrastination? "Eat that frog!" I don't mean that literally, but this is a technique that author and success expert, Brian Tracy introduced in order to effectively stop procrastination. According to him, what you need to do is eat the ugliest and most disgusting-looking frog first. What he means is that you should tackle the most challenging task first, because anything that you will do after that task will be much easier once you've gotten the hardest one out of the way. Tracy believes that with this technique, you not only beat procrastination, but it could also improve your productivity at work.

Manage Distractions

Emails, phone calls, instant messages, and even the desire to browse your social media account are some of the distractions that you face every day at work. These things add to the pressure that you're already facing while doing your job. While some of these interruptions are unavoidable, what you can do is prioritize when and how you respond to the distraction. For example, if you receive an email that doesn't need your immediate response, hold off on it until you've finished what you're supposed to be doing. Or if you have a subordinate that can take calls for you, let them handle it and just focus on your task.

Don't Say Yes to Everything

Again, do not overwhelm yourself just so you can please your boss or your co-workers. When you put too much on your plate, you'll end up either stressing yourself out because of undone tasks or doing nothing at all because you're too overwhelmed with the things you have to do. Keep in mind that you can only do so much, drop the tasks that you can do away with, and stick with those you need to prioritize.

Learn to Delegate

You might not realize it, but another thing that causes you stress is that you try to finish all your tasks on your own. If the opportunity permits, let other people help you in your task. Delegate the job to your workmate who you think is best to do the job.

Stop Controlling Everything

You just have to accept that you cannot control everything. Whenever you put pressure on yourself to make sure that things go your way, you end up stressing yourself out even more. Stop wasting your time and energy by trying to manage things that are beyond your control.

Arrive in the Office Earlier

Running late for work could cause you a lot of stress. Because you decided to stay a little bit longer in bed, you end up cutting traffic and rushing towards your office so that you won't be late. Try getting up a little bit earlier to arrive at least 15 minutes from the office to save yourself from the hassle and stress of being late.

Plus, another advantage of arriving early is that you have a few minutes of solitude in your office before everybody arrives and you start doing your daily grind.

Take Quick, Short Breaks

Do you think that working straight hours and skipping lunch and coffee breaks makes you more productive? Think again. In fact, according to experts, having a breather, even for a short five minutes, is important in order to refresh your brain and your energy. Have a quick coffee break or walk outside for a few minutes if you can and you'll see that you're more focused when you go back to your desk.

Make Friends at Work

You cannot last long in a work environment if you're a lone wolf. Create connections in your office and make friends with those who you think could give you support whenever you need it. Your work friends are the ones who understand you and who will be there for you whenever you need to release stress from work. Be sure that you're there to reciprocate by also listening to them and lending a helping hand when they need it.

Leave Everything at the Office

This is probably hard to do for most people because you will always have the itch to think about work or check your work email, even if you're already at home. However, if you really want to manage your work-related stress, you must learn how to shut down anything that has to do with work when you arrive home. That way, you will be able to shift your focus and energy to your spouse or your children.

Chapter 19: Keep A Pet

Keeping a pet is one way of reducing stress and it is proven that animals' company is cathartic especially when one is faced with emotional adversity.

Animals are a good source of companionship; they are loyal and non judgmental their love and acceptance is unconditional. Your pet will always listen to you and provide company when one would otherwise be living alone. Your fears and anxieties are easier to deal with since your pet can act as a distraction to the lingering negative thoughts.

Be sure that your pet will help you keep active and have you focus your energy on them instead of worrying. The process of taking care of your pet, going on walks and playing with them will make you active and happier. Caring for others is a big positive emotional booster, which ultimately leaves you more relaxed and in high spirits.

Pets are relaxing and keep you from thinking of or ruing your situation; you become happier more self confident and cope better when you are not bogged down by thoughts of problems. These animals can also make you alter your unhealthy behaviors; you will have to spend less time in working or at the pub so that you run home to cater to your pet.

Animals just make us happy, don't they? Pets are a welcome presence in our lives; when we are happy we have lower blood pressure and experience less tension. Scientific studies have found out that those who keep pets have a lower blood rate even while performing straining mental activities.

Pets will also help you recover quicker when you are recovering from illnesses; the mere presence of the animal is a big boost to your health and wellbeing. Since animals are touchy and feely the benefits are further increased; touch has great healing powers by reducing the production of stress hormones and stimulating the production of white blood cells to improve your body's immunity.

Why don't you try keeping a pet? It will do you a lot of good in your struggle against persistent stress. Animals are great loving companions that will bring to your life more happiness.

Take A Vacation

Sometimes it is alright to 'run away' from your problems and spend two, three or more weeks on holiday. Book your vacation and leave as soon as you can because you will feel much better when you get there; you will be happier and will come back highly charged and reinvigorated.

Taking a vacation has numerous benefits for your emotional and social wellbeing; it improves your health and emotional balance. Holidays are great fighters of everyday stress and it does not have to be long; it allows you to detach from familiar stress triggering environments like our jobs for mental relaxation and emotional boosting.

Make sure that you plan and research your vacation well so that you are not hounded by travel stress; take care of your travel, accommodation at the destination and do not forget to leave your house in order. Take care of everything at home and at work before you leave so that you are not bothered while on vacation with more stress.

When you get away from stressful environments, chances of contracting cardio vascular problems like heart disease are reduced considerably. Production of toxic stress hormones is cut off immediately you leave a stress pot and in addition, holidays are a lot of fun thus triggering feel good hormones which helps counter the effects of stress.

You will be energized and more focused after your vacation, with less chances of illness which you would otherwise be prone to due to the damage caused by stress hormones to your immune system.

Another part of our lives that will cause us immense stress is a dysfunctional sex life. Stress is a direct contributor to diminished libido, however regular vacationers have reported improved sex lives, feel sexier and are more romantic. When your sex life is healthy you will have high self confidence and less stressed.

Vacationing makes you happier leaving you with feeling good, less anxious or nervous with a general feeling of well being. When you go on vacation with your partner or children, your relationship will be strengthened and bring you closer.

Try vacationing for stress management and be assured that you will return a better, happier, reinvigorated person. Holidays are great for your health.

Chapter 20: Take Control Of Your Environment

If you are stressed, the best thing you can do is try to maintain control of your surroundings. When you don't have control over your environment, thing can get messy really quickly. There are a lot of things you can do to help defuse a stressful situation. Below is a list of things you can do to control or change a stressful situation.

Share your feelings. It is hard for other people to know what you are feeling if you don't tell them. And if people don't understand what the problem is, how can they help to fix it?

Be willing to compromise. Maybe it can't be the way you wanted but there has to be a middle ground that is ok. Most people are willing to compromise if they are given the chance.

Manage your time. If your stress is caused by time management problems, you will need to learn to manage your time more efficiently. This is a situation that is totally up to you to fix.

Learn to accept the things that you cannot change and move on. Also recognize the things that you can change, and then change them.

Forgive easily. One of the best things you can give yourself is the power to forgive others. Its will free you from regret and guilt.

Try to always see the positive in every situation even if it seems like there isn't one. People who can always see the good in any situation tend to be a lot happier.

Reduce the intensity of your emotions. If you are emotionally all over the place, other people will be too. It will only serve to elevate the situation. If you can control your emotions or just lessen them, it will help others do the same.

Get organized. If you are organized, it will automatically reduce stress. There will be less to worry about and stress over. You don't have to wonder where things are or how you will get things done if it is organized.

Learn to accept yourself and others. We all have flaws; no one is perfect. Accepting that will help you understand yourself and others better.

Don't push yourself too hard. There is only so much you can handle at once. Pace your self, others will understand.

While this is just a short list of the things you can do to control your environment, it is a great place to start. Being in control will lessen the stress that you feel. It will also with relieving the stress of people around you. When you are in control, other people will feel safer and the situation will be easier to deal with.

Making Time For Yourself

You need to have time for yourself. It can be a few minutes or a whole day. Because you cannot put more hours into your day, you need to use time management. Your mental health is just as important if not more important than your physical health.

Do something that you love everyday.

The first step to making time for yourself is deciding that you deserve it. Stop feeling guilty or selfish for doing things that make you happy. This time should be completely dedicated to something that you love to do or things that make you happy.

During your time, do not do things for other people. Only do things that will make you happy and help you relax. It is ok to say no. You do things for other all of the time and it's ok to take care of yourself. You need it and you are worth it.

Even if you day seems like it is completely full make sure that you take the time to assess where you are at mentally and to relax. You can only be your best self when you are relaxed and reduce your stress. It is not selfish to make time for you. You can start by making a list of how you spend your day. After you have the list it will be easy to see where there is room to make time for yourself.

Make a list of fun or relaxing things that you would like to do. This can be a list of things that you know you like or you can add things that you have thought about doing but have not had the chance to do yet.

When you are making your schedule, make sure to add time for yourself. Treat it like it is a meeting or an appointment that you need to keep. When you have your free time do things from your list. The things on your list should be things that make your feel refreshed and relaxed. Read that book that you have been putting off. Take a walk in the park. It doesn't matter what it is as long as you are doing something for you.

Most of us spend so much time doing things for others that we forget that we matter too. If you are too stressed to help yourself, how will you be able to help the people that need you?

Making time for yourself to do the things that make you happy and to do the things you love to do will help make you more motivated in your daily life. You will end up getting more done overall. When you are happy, even the tasks that you don't want to do will seem easier.

Chapter 21: Healthy Habits That Beat Stress

In the previous chapters of this book, we discussed how stress can affect one's health and wellbeing. I hope by now you've realized that your habits are one of the main reasons why you experience stress. In order to cope with stress and avoid its perilous effects, what you need to do is practice healthy habits that lead you to ultimately beat stress.

Keep a Routine

Routines are important because they make daily life easy since you already have a "structure" to follow. It's like you're running an automatic vehicle in which you are able to accomplish things at a certain period of time flawlessly. For example, your morning routine is to run five miles, then have breakfast, prepare, and go to work; when afternoon comes, your routine is to have a break and check your email; in the evening, your routine is having dinner with the family and enjoying reading a good book before you turn in for the day. With this routine you were able to eat three whole meals, exercise, go to work, and have time for you and your family, which creates the work-life balance that you need in order to reduce stress in your life.

Exercise

Don't miss the chance to engage in physical activity, especially when you're stressed. Research has shown that regular exercise can actually reduce the effects of both mental and physical stress. Individuals who had regular physical activity were seen to have a lower risk of developing anxiety and depression. Cardio exercises like running, swimming, or spinning do not only help you lose weight and improve your heart's health, but it also has stress-busting benefits too.

Have a 1-on-1 with a Person You Trust

You're like a ticking bomb if you have the habit of keeping your feelings to yourself.

That's why it's important that you have someone whom you trust that will listen to you vent your negative emotions and at the same time give you words of encouragement and support. Call your best friend, your mom, talk to your partner, and share with them your thoughts, your worries, and your triumphs. This will surely be a good dose of medicine to manage stress.

Get Quality Sleep

Remember how irritable and groggy you are when you don't get enough sleep? Not only does sleep deprivation limit your focus and impact your mood, it also increases your stress levels and anxiety as well. Try to get at least seven hours of sleep daily and see how it helps you better manage your stress.

Always Say "Thank You"

Showing gratitude by saying "thank you" or doing an act of random kindness has been found to help reduce anxiety. Try practicing gratitude as soon as you open your eyes—be thankful for what you have: your job, your family, your home, etc. Doing this will ensure that you're set for a great day ahead.

Allot Time to Disconnect

Set the most convenient time when you will just sit comfortably in a corner to enjoy the solitude. Get rid of your mobile phone, email, or TV, and just relish the silence. Use this time to reflect, pray, or meditate. Research show that disconnecting from all the clutter and noise will help reduce stress levels and tension in the body.

Quit Smoking and Excessive Drinking

Whenever you're stressed, do you tend to light a cigarette, believing that it will help reduce your stress? Or do you ask your friends for a night of drinking when the pressure in the office is just too much and getting drunk is your only way out? Although most smokers think that lighting a stick can help relieve their stress, in contrast to research, which shows that nicotine, in cigarette, actually increases stress hormones in the body. Not only that, research also shows that smokers have higher stress levels than non-smokers. Drinking alcohol excessively also has the same effect of increasing the production of stress hormones in the body. So if you're really serious about managing your stress, you have to be willing to give up smoking and drinking right away.

Eat Healthy Food

Did you know that the food you eat also affects your stress levels? According to health experts, there are certain types of food that can aggravate stress. Some examples of these are: fast foods, energy drinks, coffee, sodas, and food laden with sugar. Being mindful of what you put on your plate and making sure that you always eat a healthy, well-rounded meal is one of the easiest ways for you to manage your stress.

Move to the next chapter to discover foods that can help beat stress!

Conclusion

Stress is among the many factors that decreases an individual's self-esteem. When this happens, certain problems arise, like health-related problems, coping up, family problems, and a whole lot more.

Stress is felt once there is pressure from work or from doing many tasks all at once, from issues concerning relationships, money problems and in the society. Stress management is just the solution to this problem. There is a need for us to learn stress management techniques that way we may be able to learn how to handle stress effectively.

We know that we are stressed when we feel different physiological symptoms such as headache, having difficulty of sleeping, increased anxiety, losing of appetite, and having cold or a flu. There is also feelings of frustration and losing of hope.

Some individuals even experience fuzzy thinking or being absent-minded. Some forget to take care of themselves and they looked like they were stunned by a stun gun TASER because of their absent minded looks. Generally speaking, stress affects a person's whole being.

If an individual will really strive hard in order to combat stress, it is of no doubt that he will properly manage all the pressures that he faces. There are different ways in order to properly manage stress.

It will be very beneficial to know them since it will develop our coping up skills, enables us to quickly solve problems and handle every stressful situation. It may take some time to fully develop this skills but it pays off once you get to master the proper management of stress.

The main foundation of stress management is learning to take control of life. Let not stress run your life because it will only ruin your day. It is the nature of our work to become very demanding and thus making us become severely stressed and exhausted from doing so many tasks. These few tips on how to manage stress will be of great help in your everyday life.

First of all, it is important to identify the sources of your stress. This can be possible by looking at your own habits, your attitude or personality.

These are the important areas that need to be focused since they affect your ability of coping up with stress. Keeping a diary or perhaps a list of all your stressors and how you managed them will let you know what needs to be changed on your personality for you to handle stress.

Secondly, you need to evaluate yourself as to how you cope with stress. Through the list of stressors that you have, you may then be able to know whether your management skills are effective or whether it has improved your coping skills. It lets you identify more new and effective strategies to deal with stress.

Third, you can benefit from managing stress in healthy ways either you go spend some time off or have a vacation. Relaxing from time to time does not necessarily mean that you are escaping from a problem but rather it will remind you that you need to take a break and give importance to your body.

Adopting a healthy lifestyle will strengthen your physical health and it increases your resistance to stress. Engaging in activities that will give you fun and enjoyment will also make you feel at ease.

Just like rechargeable stun guns, we need to recharge ourselves and gather more energy that way we can effectively manage the different forms of stress that comes our way.

Having a relaxed mind, a healthy way of living, staying calm, and use of coping techniques such as time management and maintaining a positive attitude will all help an individual to manage his stress.

CPSIA information can be obtained
at www.ICGtesting.com
Printed in the USA
LVHW050040220221
679515LV00003B/330